Single Surgical Procedures 43

A Colour Atlas of

Transthoracic Repair of Hiatus Hernia

Robert Pringle

Ch.M, FRCS (Ed), FRCS(Eng)
Consultant Surgeon
Ninewells Hospital and Medical School
Dundee

Wolfe Medical Publications Ltd
Year Book Medical Publishers, Inc

Published by Wolfe Medical Publications, 1987
Printed by W.S. Cowell Ltd, 8 Buttermarket, Ipswich, United Kingdom

ISBN 07234 1073 9

This book is one of the titles in the series of Wolfe Single Surgical Procedures, a series which will eventually cover some 200 titles.

For a full list of Atlases in this series, plus forthcoming titles and details of our surgical, dental and veterinary Atlases, please write to Wolfe Medical Publications Ltd, Wolfe House, 3 Conway Street, London W1P 6HE
or
Year Book Medical Publishers, Inc, 35 East Wacker Drive, Chicago, Ill. 60601

Distributed in Continental North and Central America, Hawaii and Puerto Rico by Year Book Medical Publishers, Inc.

Library of Congress Cataloging in Publication Data

Pringle, Robert.
A colour atlas of transthoracic repair of hiatus hernia.

(Single surgical procedures series; v. 43)
Includes index.
1. Hiatal hernia—Surgery—Atlases. I. Title.
II. Series. [DNLM: 1. Hernia, Diaphragmatic—surgery—atlases. WF 17 P957c]
RD539.5.P75 1987 617'.559 87–15950
ISBN 0-8151-6842-X

We list below a few of the other titles in print and in preparation in the Single Surgical Procedures series. For a comprehensive list please write.

Published

Parotidectomy
Traditional Meniscectomy
Inguinal Hernias & Hydroceles in Infants and Children
Surgery for Pancreatic & Associated Carcinomata
Subtotal Thyroidectomy
Anterior Resection of Rectum
Boari Bladder-Flap Procedure
Surgery for Varicose Veins
Treatment for Carpal Tunnel Syndrome
Seromyotomy for Chronic Duodenal Ulcer
Surgery for Undescended Testes
Operations on the Internal Carotid Artery
Renal Transplant
Lumbar Discography
Visceral Artery Reconstruction
Flexor Tendon Repair
Proctocolectomy
Common Operations of the Foot
Right Hemicolectomy
Extra-cranial and Intra-cranial Anastomosis
Surgery for Hirschsprung's Disease
Thyroid Lobectomy
Surgery at the Thoracic Outlet
External Fixation
Anterior Cervical Spine Fusion
Liver Transplantation
Modified Radical Mastectomy
Paratopic Transplant of Body and Tail of the Pancreas
Subdiaphragmatic Total Gastrectomy for Malignant Disease
Rupture of the Rotator Cuff
Left Hemicolectomy
Cleft Lip Surgery
Gastric Revision Operations
Plastering Techniques
Congenital Dislocation of Hip
Mastectomy with Immediate Reconstruction
Joint Replacement of Wrist and Hand

In Production

Joint Replacement of the Hand
Periodontal Surgery

Some Future Titles

Biliary Enteric Anastomosis with Strictures in Common Bile Duct
Surgical Disencumberment of the Thoracic Outlet
Aortic Endarterectomy
Axillary Dissection for Melanoma
Groin Dissection for Melanoma
Coronary Artery Bypass
Omental Transposition
Orthopaedic Hip Approaches
Management of Venous Disease
Upper Thoracic Sympathectomy
Inguinal Hernia Repair
Vascular Access
Dental Analgesia
Hiatus Hernia
Plastic and Reconstructive Surgery
Occlusion/Malocclusion
Femoral and Tibial Osteotomy
Resection of Aortic Aneurysm
Ileo-Rectal Anastomosis
Techniques of Nerve Grafting and Repair
Surgery for Dupuytren's Contracture
Athrodesis of the Ankle
Spondylolisthesis
Repair of Prolapsed Rectum
Splendectomy
Anterior Nephrectomy
Caecocystoplasty
Billroth 1 Gastroectomy
Billroth 2 Gastroectomy
Abdominal Incisions
Throacotomy
Appendicectomy
Incisional Hernia
Lung Lobectomy
Lung Removal
Haemorrhoids
Rectosigmoid Resection
Surgery for Anorectal Incontinence
Visceral Vascular Occlusion
Aortofemoral Bypass
Aortoilac Dtsobliteration

General Editor, Wolfe Surgical Atlases:
William F. Walker, DSc, ChM, FRCS (Edin. and England), FRS (Edin.). Professor of Clinical Surgery at the University of Dundee.

Contents

Acknowledgements

I am grateful to Dr W. I. K. Bisset for the section on anaesthetic management and for his professional skills, patience and enthusiasm.

I am also indebted to Mr Tom King, Head of the Medical Illustration Service Ninewells Hospital and Medical School, and his staff, for the photographs and for their helpfulness and courtesy.

Introduction

The commonest type of hernia through the oesophageal hiatus is the sliding or Type I hernia (80%). In this variety the gastrooesophageal junction lies above the diaphragm and reflux of gastric content almost always occurs and indeed is responsible for the oesophagitis and its sequelae. The paraoesophageal hernia or Type II (15%) exists when a variable amount of the fundus and greater curvature of the stomach herniate through the hiatus into the chest. In this variety the gastrooesophageal junction is situated in its normal position below the diaphragm and reflux is uncommon. Incarceration and strangulation are known complications. The mixed, or Type III, hernia (5%) occurs when almost all of the stomach has herniated into the thoracic cavity. The gastrooesophageal junction in this variety can lie either above or below the diaphragm and it follows that reflux may or may not be present. This hernia is also liable to incarceration and strangulation. Rarely, other structures may be present in the Type III hernia, such as colon or small bowel in addition to the stomach. This variation has been called a Type IV hernia.

Diagnosis

A thorough history and physical examination followed by a Barium swallow and meal, together with oesophagoscopy, are the basic investigations required for diagnosis. Proper evaluation of the symptoms and findings is necessary before deciding on treatment. **Since most of the symptoms of a sliding hiatus hernia are due to the reflux oesophagitis associated with the hernia, then it follows that endoscopy is the most important step in the diagnosis. The radiological finding of a sliding hernia is not sufficient in itself to justify operation**. If oesophagitis is not present on oesophagoscopy then the patient's symptoms may be due to another cause.

Occasionally reflux is found at radiological examination without evidence of a hernia and in these circumstances operation is sometimes necessary if the patient's symptoms are severe enough and if conservative therapy has failed.

Ischaemic heart disease, biliary colic and peptic ulceration can mimic the symptoms of a hernia and can lead to diagnostic confusion. Unfortunately, any combination of these conditions can exist and fine clinical judgement is required to give proper weighting to the patient's symptoms. In these complex cases one may have to proceed to other investigations such as oesophageal manometry, pH telemetry, acid infusion tests, oesophageal clearance studies and investigation of the biliary tract, combined with a sound cardiological assessment, before coming to a final conclusion as to the most appropriate treatment for the individual patient.

Indications for operation

In cases of sliding hiatus hernia, a period of conservative management is desirable in the first instance. If this fails then operation should be advised to avoid the development of late complications such as anaemia and stricture. If there are no contraindications to operation because of the patient's general medical status all other types of hiatus hernia should be operated on when first diagnosed. This is because of the dangers of incarceration and strangulation. It is, unfortunately, only too common for patients to be referred for operation when they are too old and frail for a major surgical procedure. Such patients often give a history going back many years and should have been referred for operation much earlier.

The development of chronic anaemia from blood loss, in a patient who is being managed conservatively, is an indication for operation. **If the patient is shown to be developing a stricture or if oesophagitis persists in spite of intensive conservative management, then operation should be undertaken**. Many patients with reflux have repeated attacks of respiratory infection due to aspiration occurring during the night—**operation is required in these patients**.

Choice of operation

The number of operations described for the repair of a hiatus hernia serves to emphasize the controversy which existed about the nature of the mechanism which prevents reflux of gastric juice into the lower oesophagus. Although this controversy has not been completely resolved, the increasing awareness of the anatomical and physiological factors involved has led to fewer operations. Only those which attempt to correct these abnormalities have any hope of lasting success and acceptance. **The essential requirements are that the oesophagus must be sufficiently mobilised to enable the gastrooesophageal junction and 3–4 cm of oesophagus to lie within the abdominal cavity**. This intra-abdominal oesophagus should be partially surrounded by the fundus of the stomach and there should be an oblique angle of entry of the lower end of the oesophagus into the stomach. The operation gradually evolved by Belsey fulfils all these criteria and this is the operation which, in my opinion and that of many surgeons, is the operation of choice in most circumstances. **If the hiatus hernia is complicated by an organic stricture, then the patient will require a more extensive procedure involving a resection of the stricture and some form of oesophageal reconstruction or replacement**.

Preoperative preparation

A thorough history should be taken, and a physical examination performed in all cases. A preoperative ECG and chest xray, urea and electrolytes are mandatory and any abnormalities found should be assessed and treated. Anaemia should be corrected prior to surgery and if blood transfusion is required it should take place at least 48 hours **before** operation. In most cases two units of blood ought to be adequate for replacement during operation and in the immediate postoperative period.

The patient's pulmonary function must be ascertained, preoperative physiotherapy undertaken and, **where necessary**, appropriate antibiotic therapy should be instituted. A detailed explanation of the operation and the reasons for it are basic steps in getting the patient's informed consent for the operation. If it is thought that the patient will require respiratory support in an intensive care unit for a few hours postoperatively, it is my practice to introduce the intensive care team to the patient. Such measures help to ensure the patient's co-operation and go a considerable way to allay his fears.

Anaesthetic management

Patients undergoing this operation require careful preoperative preparation, as already detailed. Considerable expertise and a high standard of care are required by the anaesthetist to provide optimum operating conditions and minimise the complications that can occur. These patients are often in their sixties and seventies and suffering from other chronic medical conditions.

Surgical access is greatly helped by collapsing the left lung during operation, using a double lumen endobronchial tube such as a Robertshaw. **ECG monitoring throughout is essential and invasive intra-arterial monitoring is highly desirable.** The latter allows continuous recording of blood pressure alterations and, through intermittent sampling, also measures blood gas changes. Active warming of the patient by a thermostatically controlled water blanket and capnometry to provide continuous end tidal carbon dioxide monitoring are also useful adjuncts. **Anaesthesia can be carried out in a safe and adequate manner, however, using a standard orotracheal tube and noninvasive methods of monitoring blood pressure.**

Premedication is a matter of personal choice. Either a benzodiazepine or an intramuscular narcotic allows the patient to arrive in the theatre in a calm and co-operative state.

After establishing a secure intravenous drip, preferably in the left arm, the patient should be preoxygenated to allow optimal intubating conditions for the passage of the Robertshaw endobronchial tube. **As there is a risk of regurgitation from oesophageal reflux, intubation should be performed using Sellick's manoeuvre following an intravenous induction.** Initial profound relaxation is gained with the short acting relaxant Suxamethonium Chloride. A left-sided Robertshaw is easier to position correctly as the right-sided version has to be placed very accurately to avoid blockage of the right apical bronchus. **On inflation of the tube cuffs, particular care must be taken to check that both lungs can be inflated together and independently. The need for excessive inflation pressure is a sign of faulty positioning and can produce a tension pneumothorax if not corrected.** If after repositioning, satisfactory conditions cannot be obtained, the tube should be removed and the right-sided version tried. If still unsuccessful, attempts should be abandoned and an ordinary orotracheal tube inserted.

Anaesthesia is maintained using a long-acting competitive relaxant, nitrous oxide and oxygen supplemented by Isoflurane or Halothane. **Isoflurane is more cardiovascularly stable and less likely to cause dysrhythmias.** Intravenous analgesic supplementation with Fentanyl or other narcotic is also of considerable benefit in obtunding harmful nociceptive reflexes.

On positioning the patient in the modified right lateral position as shown (Figures **1** and **2**), the tube should again be checked to exclude movement resulting in faulty positioning. When required, the left lung is collapsed, and the inspired oxygen concentration is increased to at least 50% to compensate for hypoxia resulting from the altered lung ventilation/perfusion. **It is of great benefit to check the blood gases at this stage to ensure adequate ventilation.** Capnometry, if available, is also useful as a noninvasive method of checking ventilation. **Careful intraoperative monitoring of the ECG and blood pressure throughout is essential to diagnose the dysrhythmias and hypotension that can occur during surgical intervention in this area. Blood loss should be recorded throughout and replaced as required.** At the end of the procedure full reinflation of the lungs is carried out under direct vision and pleural drainage inserted and established.

Adequate control of postoperative pain resulting from the thoracotomy and pleural drain wounds accelerates a smooth post-operative recovery.

Stabilisation of the sectioned ribs at closure significantly reduces postoperative analgesic requirements and may minimise the risk of subsequent intercostal neuralgia developing. If this is supplemented by regular narcotic sedation postoperatively, adequate pain relief can be produced. **Insertion of an intercostal block with 0.5% Marcaine with 1 in 200,000 Adrenaline at the appropriate level prior to closure, and later repeated percutaneously as required, can produce excellent immediate postoperative pain relief.** Long-term reversible intercostal blocks can be produced by cryoprobing the appropriate nerves at the time of operation but there is a slight risk of producing a dysaesthesia in the occasional patient.

Other alternative methods are the use of thoracic epidurals employing the use of catheter-infused narcotics or local anaesthetics. These methods, though very successful, should only be used where skilled continuous nursing care and 24-hour immediate anaesthetic cover are available, due to the risks of possible delayed respiratory depression or hypotension developing.

The occasional patient with pre-existing respiratory or cardiac disease will benefit from elective postoperative ventilation in an ICU. This ensures adequate oxygenation and allows the administration of sedative intravenous narcotic doses which might otherwise cause respiratory and cardiovascular depression in the spontaneously breathing subject.

Thoracotomy

1 and 2 Positioning the patient. The patient is placed in the full lateral position for a thoracotomy through the left side of the chest. The right arm is placed on an arm board fixed to the operating table and the left arm is positioned on a sling support with the elbow flexed and the forearm bound with a crepe bandage to hold the forearm firmly in place. The whole arm should be level with the left shoulder and all monitoring leads, ECG electrodes and vascular access lines should be clear of the operating field and led to the head of the table. The abdomen should lie without restriction and the diathermy plate positioned under the right hip. The patient should have a pillow placed between the legs with the right leg straight and the left leg flexed slightly at the knee. A Velcro strap or three inch adhesive strapping should be used to fix the pelvis in the right lateral position. The patient should then have a sheet placed so as to cover the lower half of the body.

CAUTION: All joints on the arm slings should be firmly tightened. Make sure no part of the patient is touching a metal surface. Finally check that the patient's position is stable and that there is no tendency to tilt forwards or backwards.

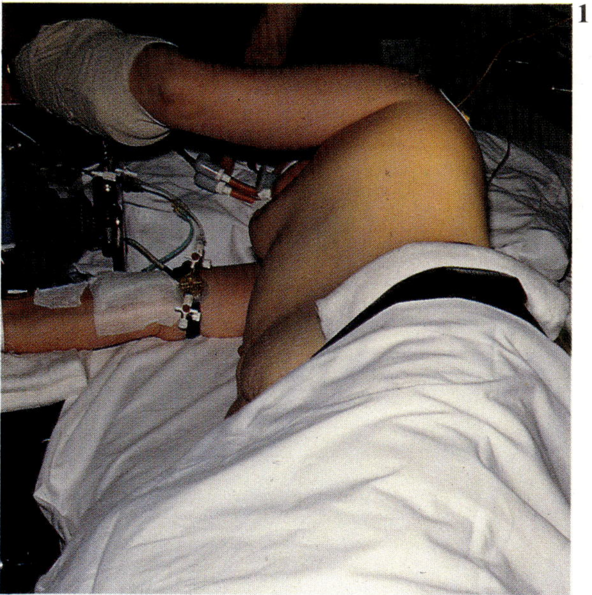

1

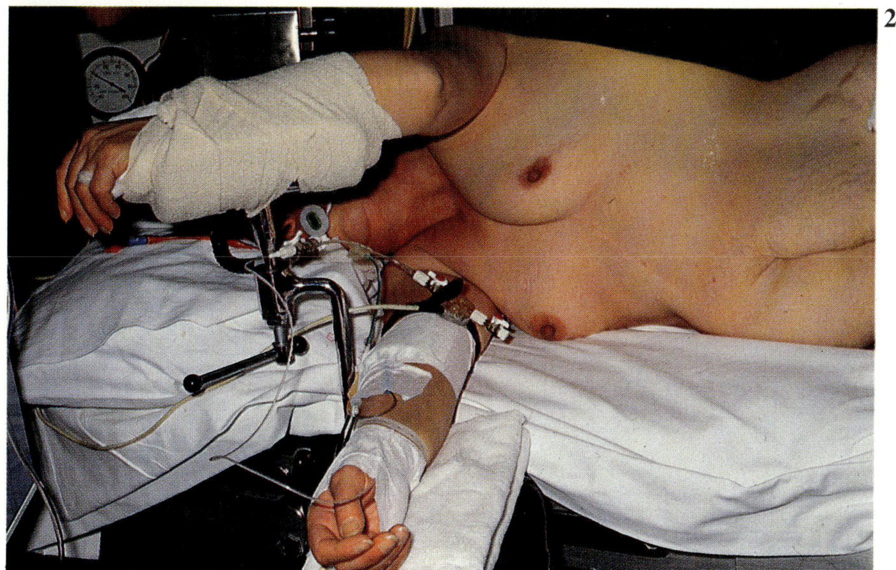

2

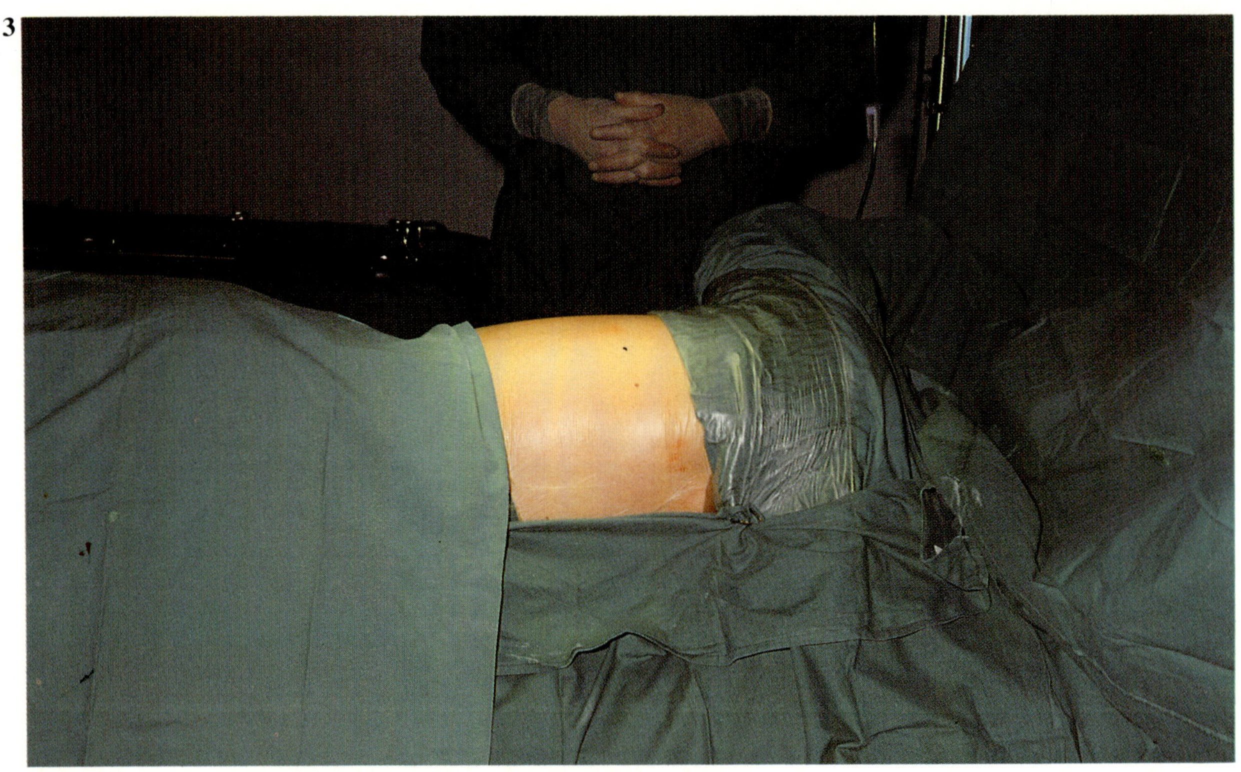

3 Preparation and towelling. The skin of the patient is prepared with two applications of Betidine antiseptic solution (Napp) from the midline anteriorly to the midline posteriorly and from the neck to the pelvis, taking care to include the left axilla, left shoulder and upper arm. The surgical solution is dried off with a dry swab and then a large sheet of Op-site or Vi-drape is applied carefully so that it covers as much as possible from midline anteriorly to midline posteriorly and from left shoulder to pelvis. Two large drapes are placed, one from the waist to cover the whole of the lower half of the patient and the other from the chest wall, below the shoulder, to cover the rest of the upper half of the patient. The top end of the latter drape can be fixed very satisfactorily by taping it to a drip stand on each side of the patient at the head of the table. One small drape is then positioned on each side joining the two large drapes so that the area of the incision is left exposed with a few inches to spare all round. The drapes are fixed in place with tetra clips or nonabsorbable stitches. The sucker nozzle, in its container, is clipped to the drapes near the left shoulder and the diathermy electrode, in its quiver, is fastened near the pelvis on the assistant's side of the table.

4 The incision. Some variation is allowable in the precise positioning of the incision but the author prefers one made over the 7th rib from the costal margin anteriorly to the paravertebral region posteriorly. If it is thought that access will be difficult then the incision can be curved upwards at its posterior end along the medial border of the scapula. After the skin incision has been made the scalpel is discarded and thereafter cutting diathermy is used throughout to divide fascia and muscle. The incision is deepened through superficial and deep fascias along the whole length of the wound.

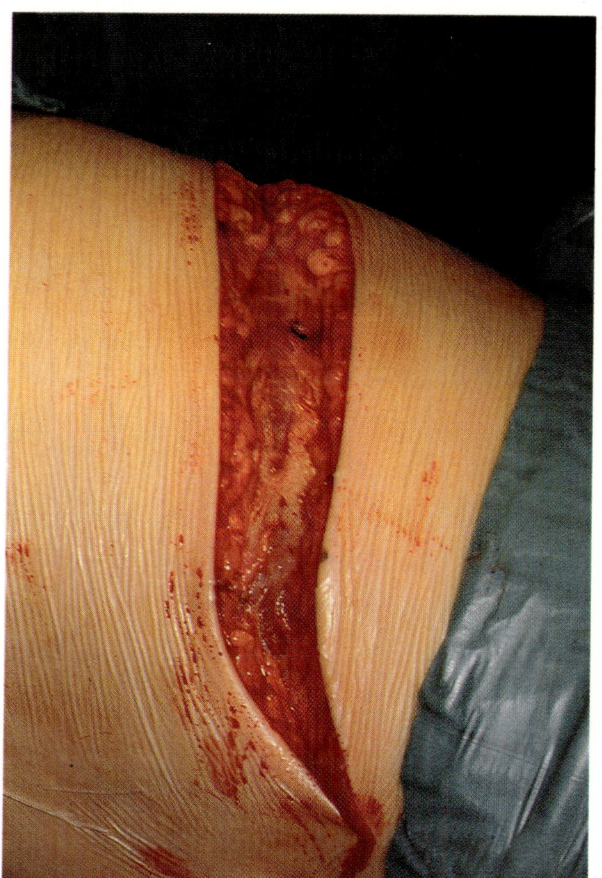

4

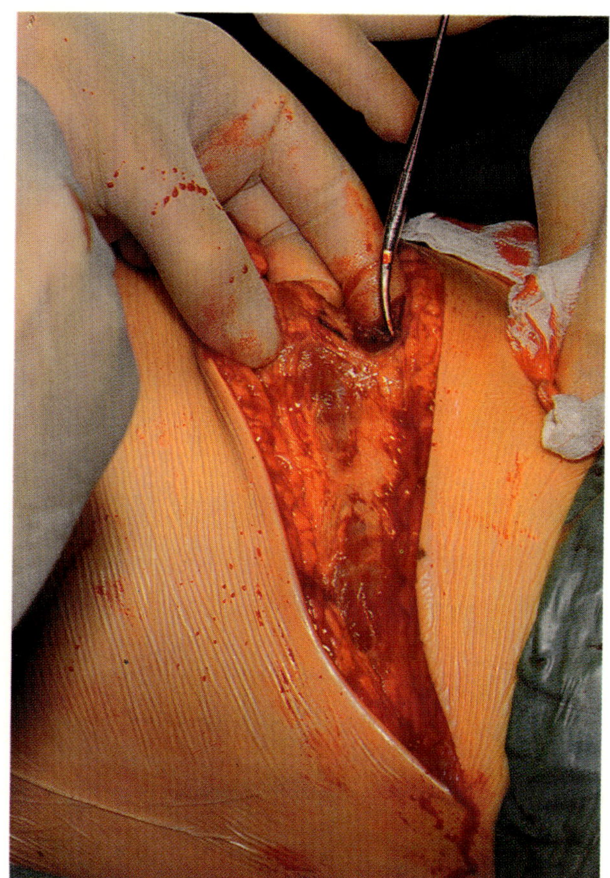

5

5 Haemostasis. Throughout the operation careful attention is paid to haemostasis. Blood loss is kept to a minimum and a dry field obtained, with the result that accurate dissection is possible. Larger vessels should be held in artery forceps and diathermied or tied using fine Nurolon. With continuous use of the diathermy the electrode has to be scraped clean with a scalpel from time to time. In the posterior part of the incision the anterior edge of the latissimus dorsi muscle is identified and the fingers are inserted under the edge of the muscle.

6

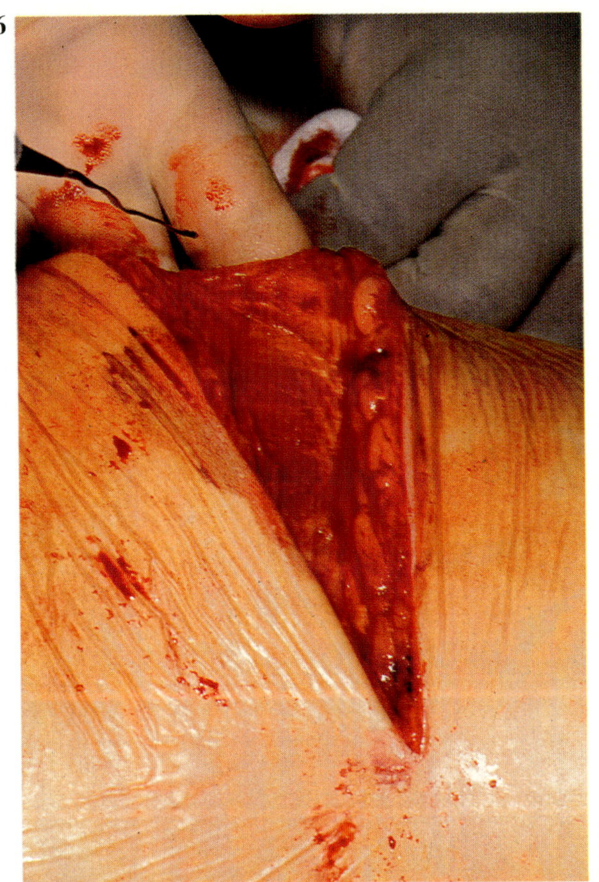

7

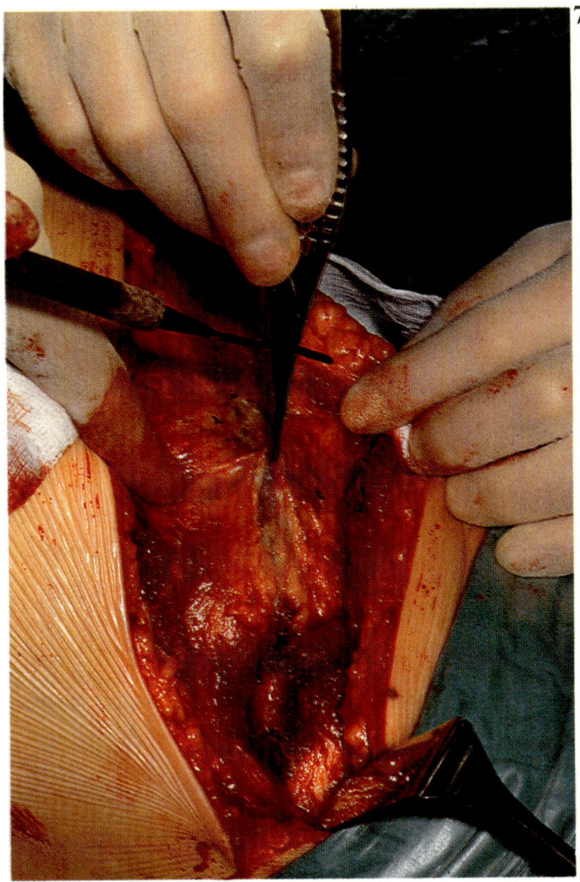

6 Division of anterior edge of latissimus dorsi. The cutting diathermy is used to divide the muscle between the opened fingers. The muscle is divided back to the posterior limit of the skin incision.

7 Diathermy of vessels. Vessels lying on the surface of the muscle should be picked up by dissecting forceps and diathermied before division of the underlying muscle.

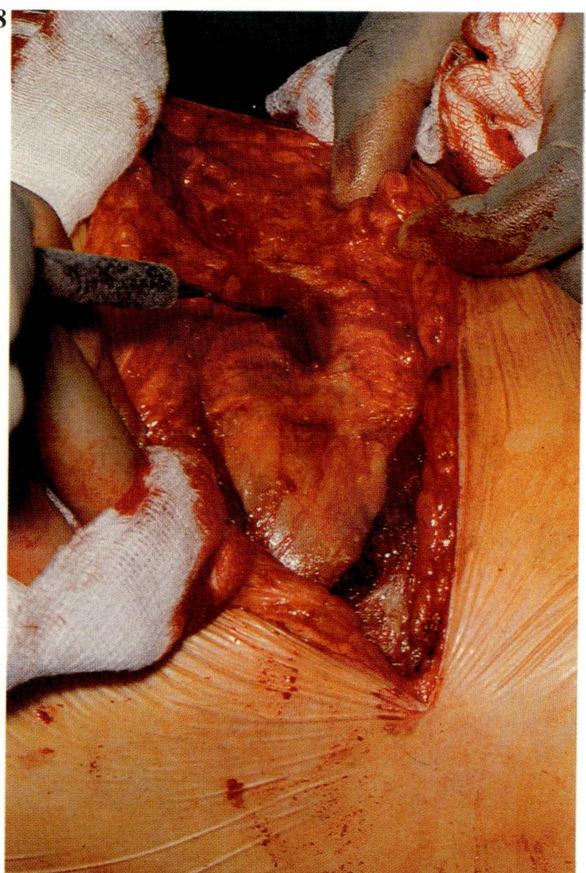

8 Exposure of serratus anterior. As the latissimus dorsi is divided the serratus anterior comes into view in the bottom of the wound.

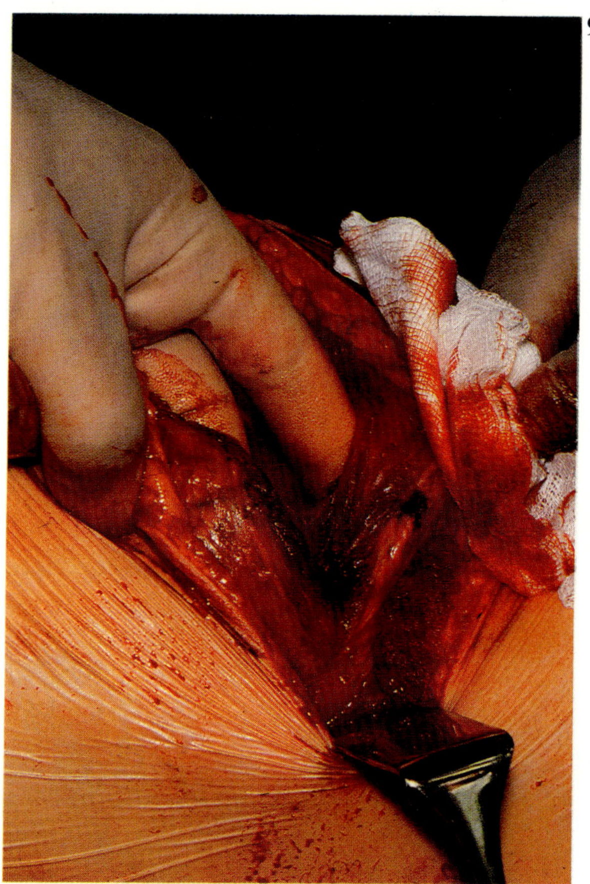

9 Exposure of rib. The serratus anterior is then divided with the fingers deep to the muscle using the cutting diathermy between the opened fingers as described before. As this division of the serratus proceeds the underlying rib can be seen coming into view in the posterior part of the incision.

10 Exposure of external oblique. As the surgeon continues along the rib in an anterior direction the fibres of the serratus anterior are found to interdigitate with those of the external oblique and the surgeon proceeds to use the diathermy to divide these fibres right down to the surface of the rib. The rib is exposed along the whole length of the incision.

At this point in the thoracotomy a decision must be made as to the final entry into the thorax. In general terms it is usual to enter the chest through the incised posterior periosteum after its mobilisation from the posterior surface for the rib. However, rigidity of the chest wall and closeness of the ribs may in some cases necessitate the complete excision of the rib for adequate access. If the chest wall is pliable some surgeons enter the thoracic cavity through an intercostal incision, leaving the ribs intact.

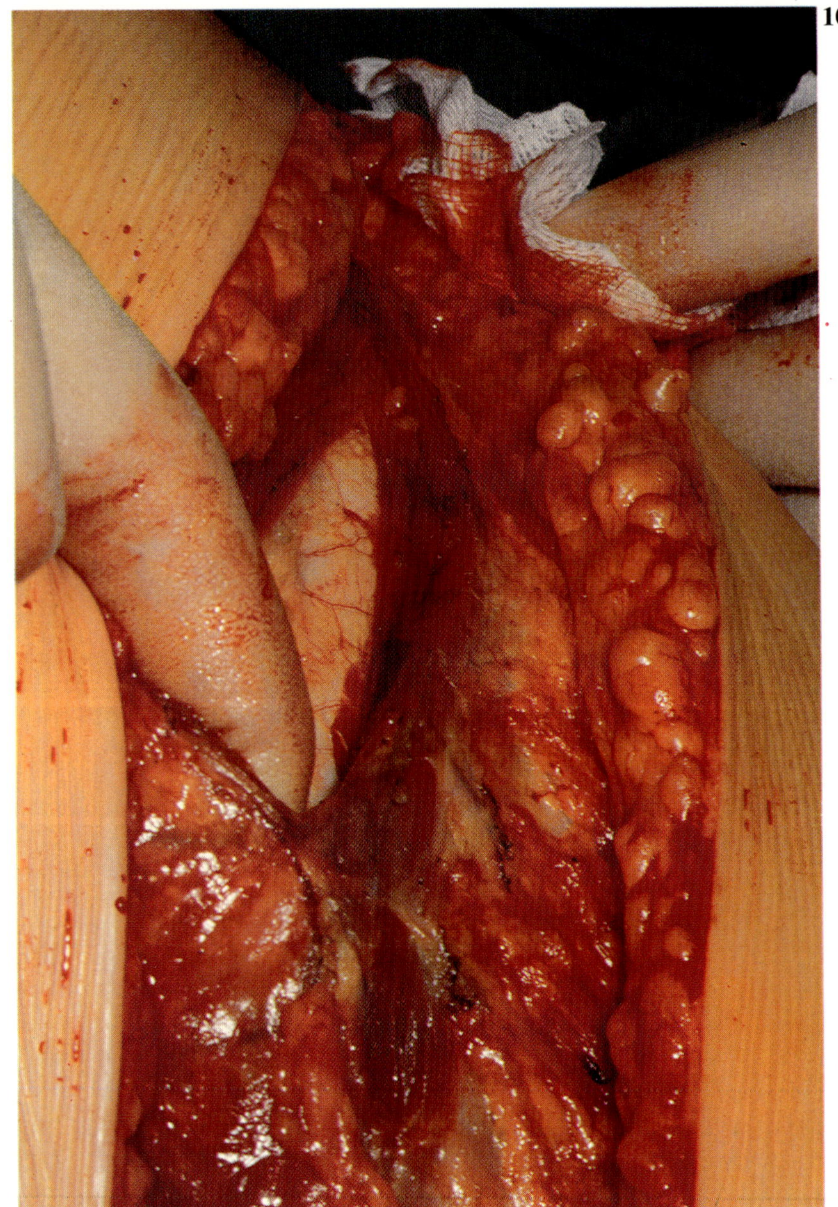
10

11

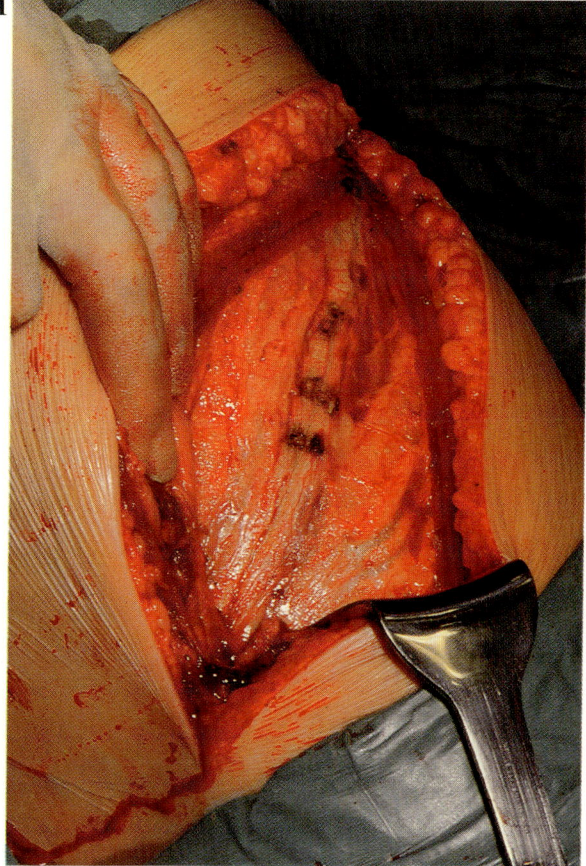

12

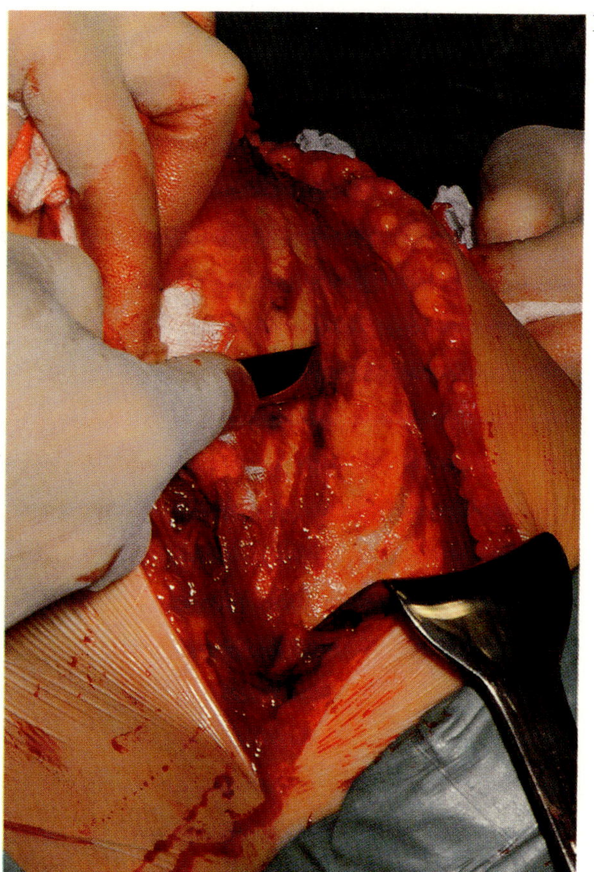

11 Incising the periosteum. Assuming that the course adopted is through the posterior periosteum, the periosteum of the rib is incised, midway between its superior and inferior borders, throughout the length of the exposed rib (using the cutting diathermy). Bleeding from the exposed rib surface is treated by diathermy coagulation. (These coagulated areas can be seen on the exposed bone)

12 Stripping the periosteum. A Tudor Edwards periosteal elevator is used to peel back the periosteum from the incised portion to the superior border of the rib along its length. It is important to take the rib clearance right to the edge of the rib and where possible over the edge.

13

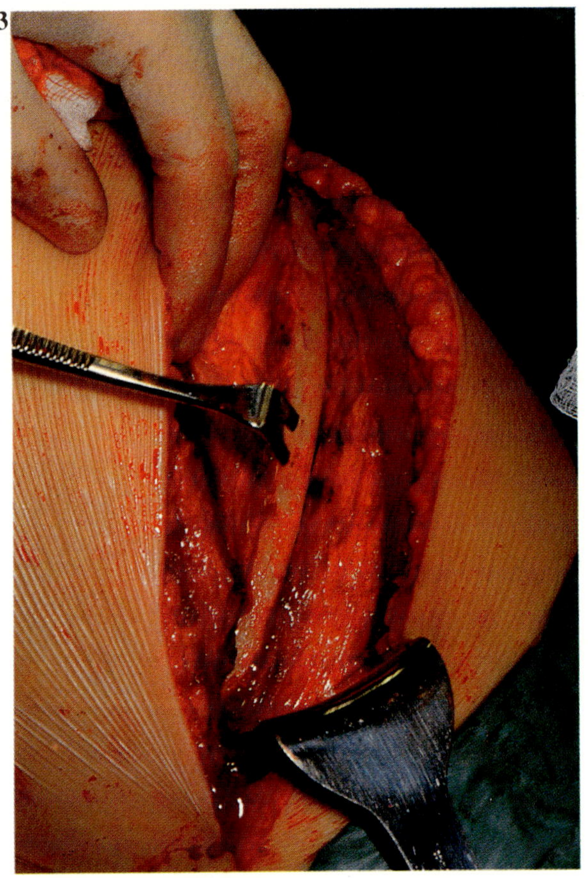

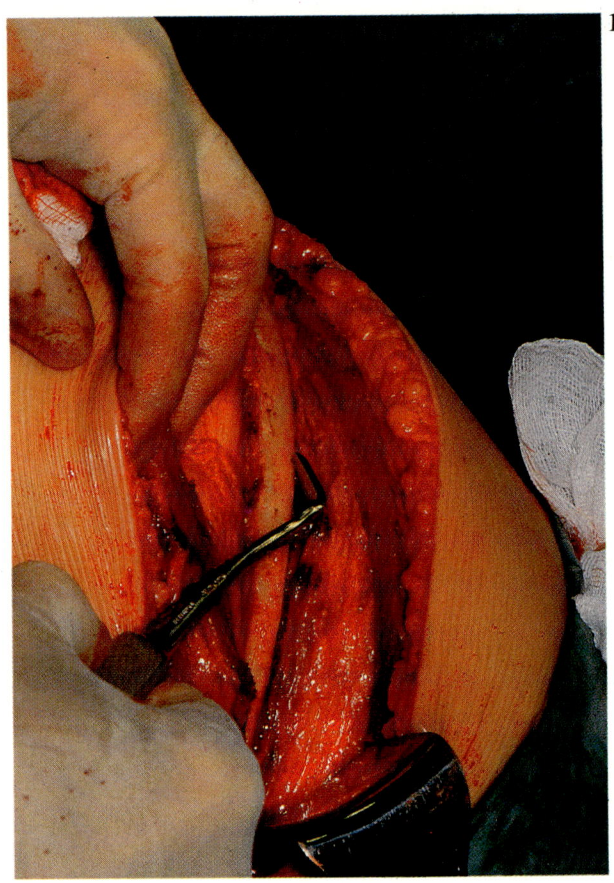

13 The rib raspatory. The Semb rib raspatory can now be used to raise the periosteum from the upper edge of the rib.

14 Detaching the intercostals. The raspatory is inserted into the defect produced by the periosteal elevator until the superior border of the rib lies in the notch of the instrument. Care is taken at this point to ensure that the instrument lies within the periosteum or else it will not strip cleanly when the raspatory is passed back and forth along the superior border of the rib. This action strips the intercostal muscles from the rib along its superior border and exposes the posterior periosteum of the rib.

15 Stripping the posterior periosteum. The periosteal elevator can be used to strip the periosteum off the posterior surface of the rib so that it appears as in this view. Note that the undamaged intercostal muscles are attached to the periosteum which has now been cleared from the anterior, the superior and the posterior part of the rib and that the posterior periosteum is exposed ready for incision into the pleural cavity. The surgeon can see the underlying lung through the pleura at this point and it is therefore possible to determine if the lung is moving freely on respiration or if it is adherent to the parietal pleura.

15

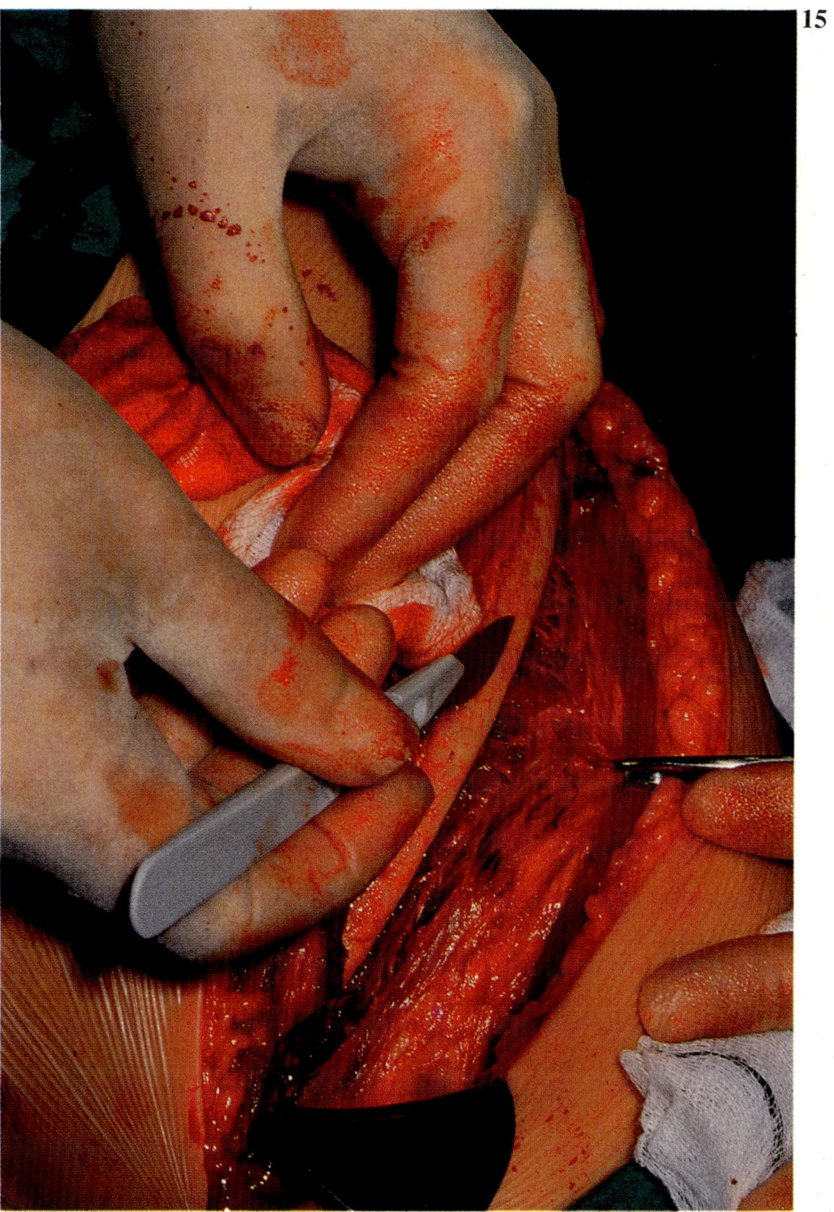

16 Entering the pleural cavity. A scalpel is now used to incise the parietal pleura. After a small opening has been made, scissors are used to extend the pleural incision along the length of the exposed posterior periosteum.

CAUTION: Take care not to damage the underlying lung, which, if it is not adherent to the parietal pleura, should fall away from the chest wall when the pleural cavity is opened.

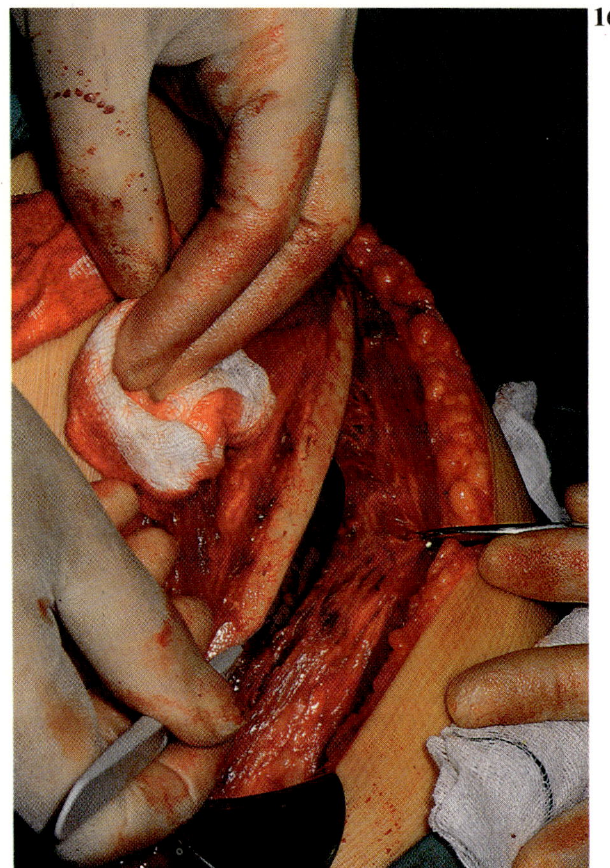

16

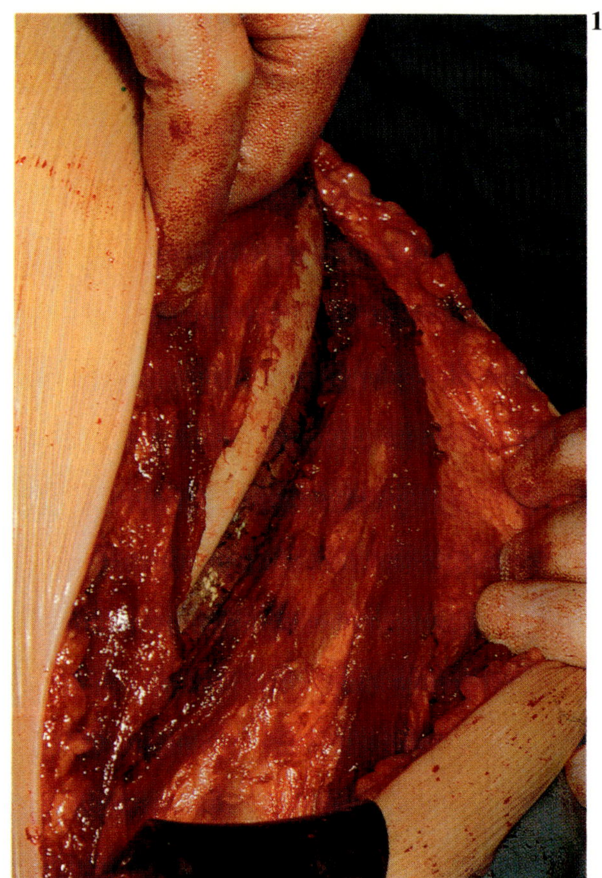

17

17 The completed incision. The thoracotomy incision is now complete and the underlying lung is visible in the depths of the wound.

18 Insertion of rib spreader. Many types of rib spreader are available but the Finochietto is the one illustrated here. The blades are inserted in the mid part of the thoracotomy wound and a few turns of the ratchet are used to open the chest incision. Initially some force is required for this but after a few minutes it is possible to perform a few more turns of the ratchet and the incision is widened until the desired exposure is achieved. If difficulty is experienced in getting enough exposure, access can be improved by dislocating the costovertebral joint of the rib posteriorly or by shearing the rib above posteriorly, after dividing the intercostal neurovascular bundle in the groove on the under surface of the rib.

CAUTION: A pack should be folded over each edge of the incision before insertion of the rib spreader in order to protect the tissues.

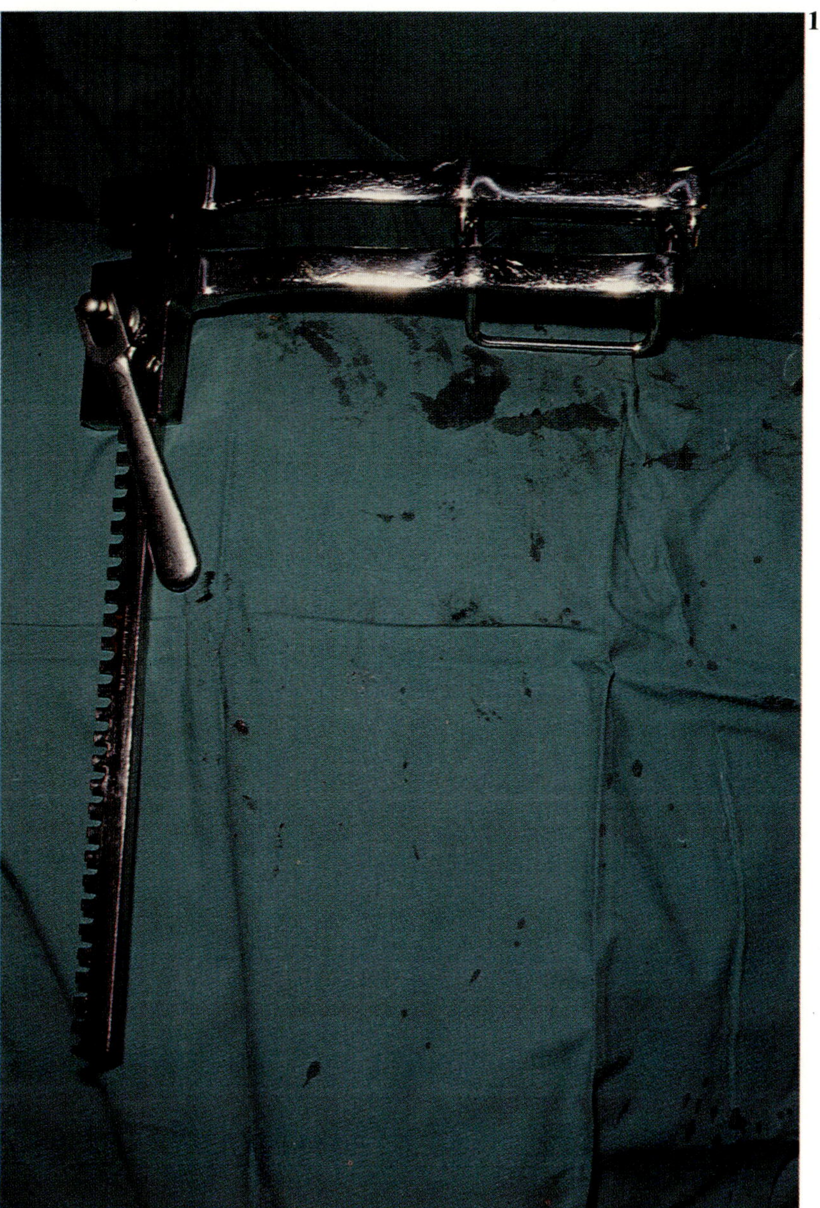

18

The antireflux procedure

19

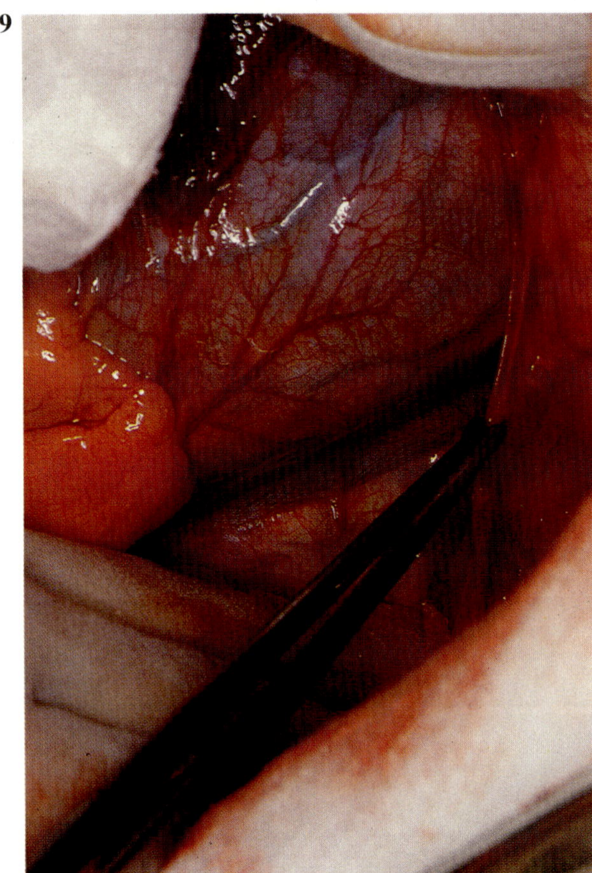

The procedure in this section is shown where possible in a slim subject so that the anatomy and operative details are easy to understand. Where indicated, the illustrations are duplicated in an obese person to demonstrate the difficulties encountered in these patients, especially for the inexperienced surgeon. The packs have been omitted in some of the illustrations to show the details of the operation without restricting the view of the operating field.

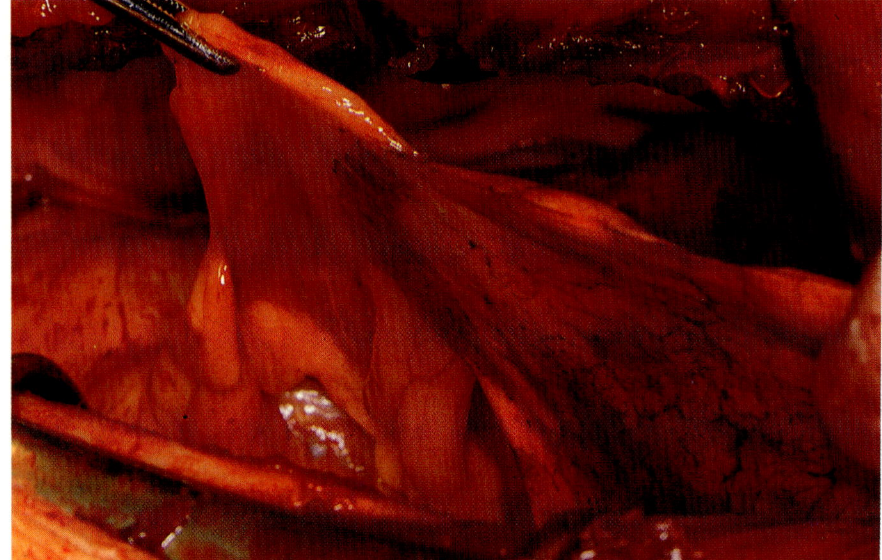

20

19 Adhesions. Adhesions are often present between the mediastinal pleura, the lung and the pericardium.

20 The same adhesions in an obese patient.

21

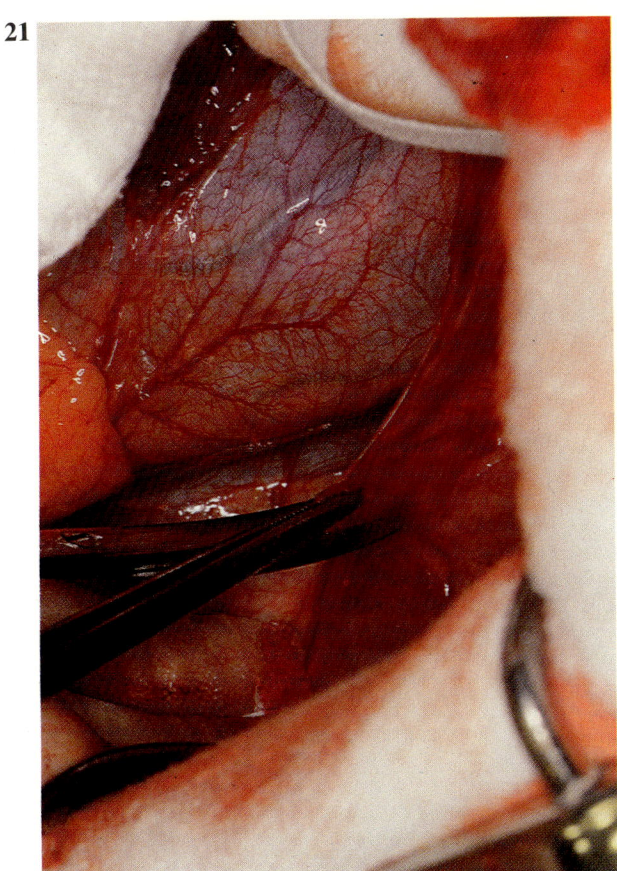

22

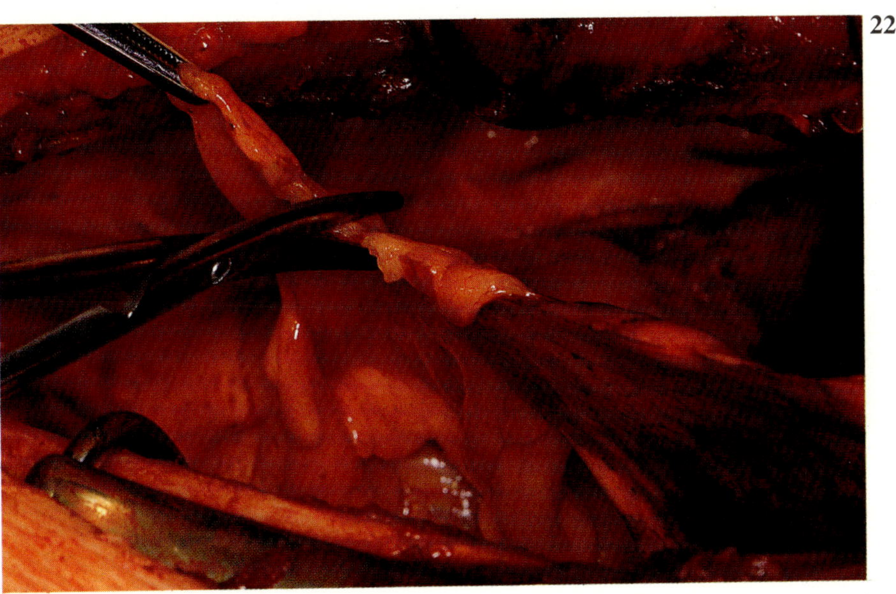

22 The same dissection in the obese patient.

21 Dissection of adhesions. These adhesions are dissected free from surrounding surfaces so that the mediastinal pleura overlying the oesophagus can be exposed.

23

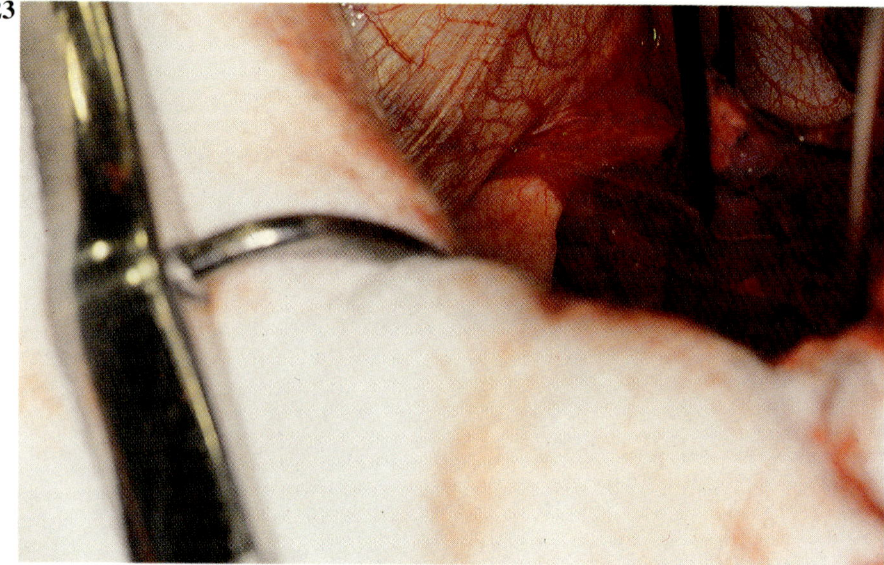

24

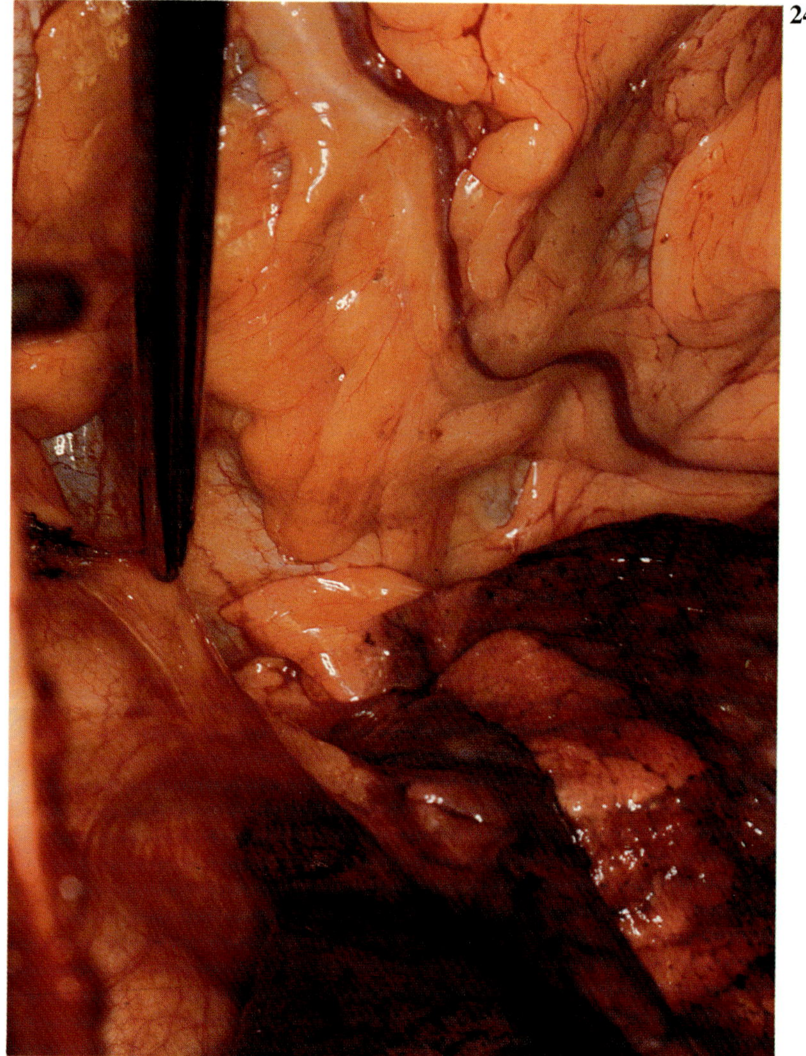

23 The pulmonary ligament. The pulmonary ligament is exposed. The adjacent lung is held away from the mediastinum in forceps to display the lower border for dissection.

24 The same view in the obese subject.

25 Division of pulmonary ligament. The pulmonary ligament is divided from its inferior margin upwards to the root of the lung.

CAUTION: Great care must be taken to avoid damaging the left pulmonary veins as the dissection proceeds upwards.

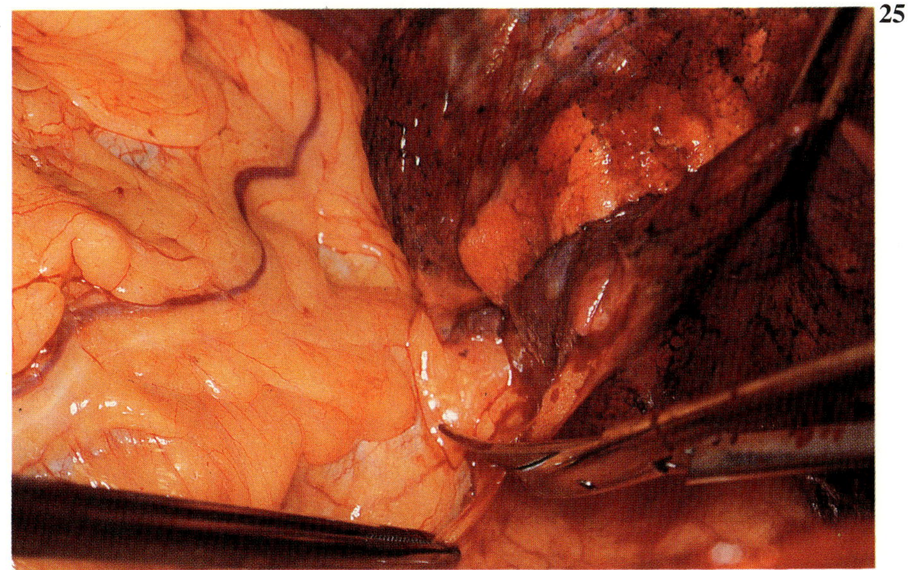

25

26 The mediastinal pleura. The mediastinal pleura overlying the lower end of the oesophagus is picked up in dissecting forceps and the pleura is dissected above as far as the root of the lung and below as far as the oesophageal hiatus to expose the oesophagus.

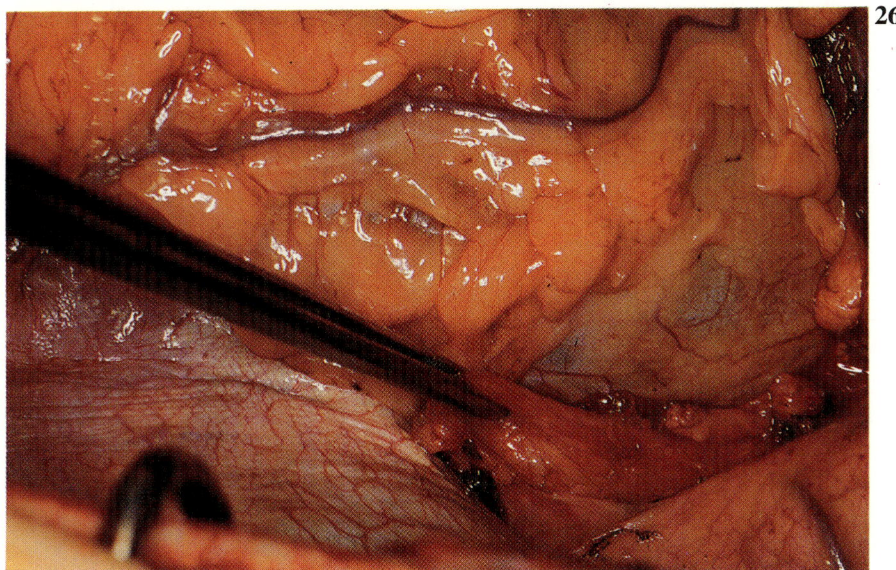

26

27 The oesophagus. The oesophagus can be seen through the opened mediastinal pleura as it comes through the hiatus, which is to the left.

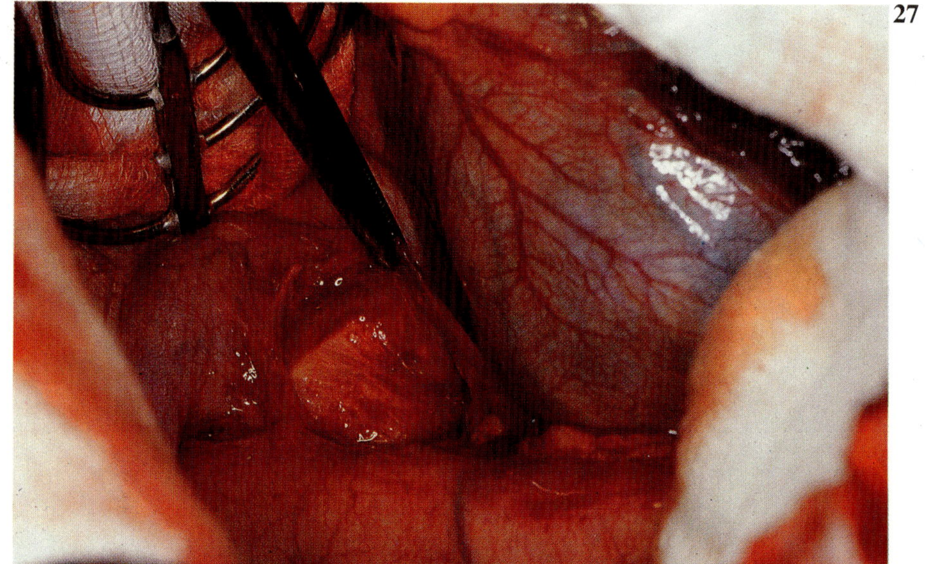

27

28 Mobilisation of the oesophagus. The oesophagus mostly lies out of sight behind the heart and is now dislocated into the left chest by, in the first instance, passing a finger behind the oesophagus.

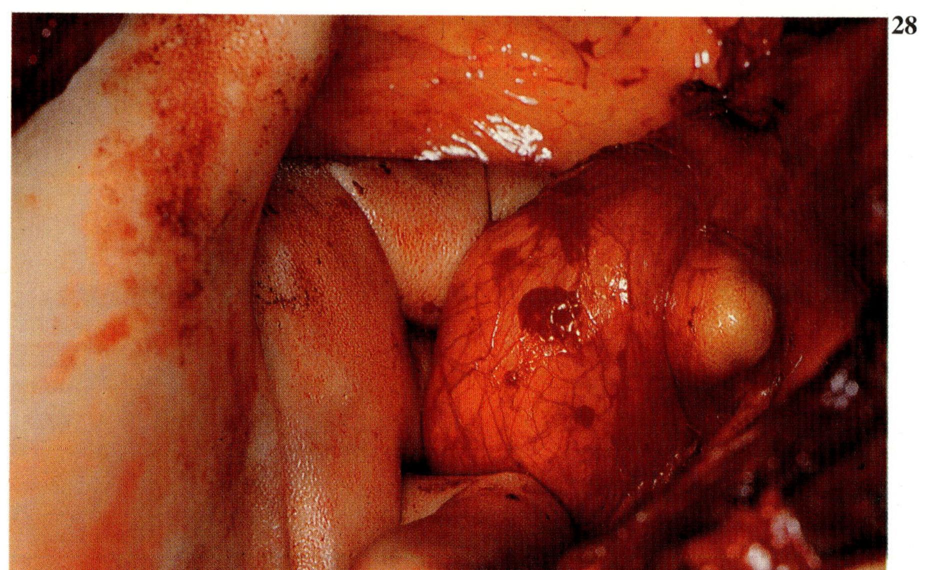

28

29 Further mobilisation of the oesophagus. Gradually insinuate another finger through the defect created until two fingers pass easily behind the oesophagus.

CAUTION: When passing the fingers behind the oesophagus it is necessary to stay as close to the oesophagus as is possible in order to avoid opening into the right pleural cavity which is in close relationship to the other side of the oesophagus.

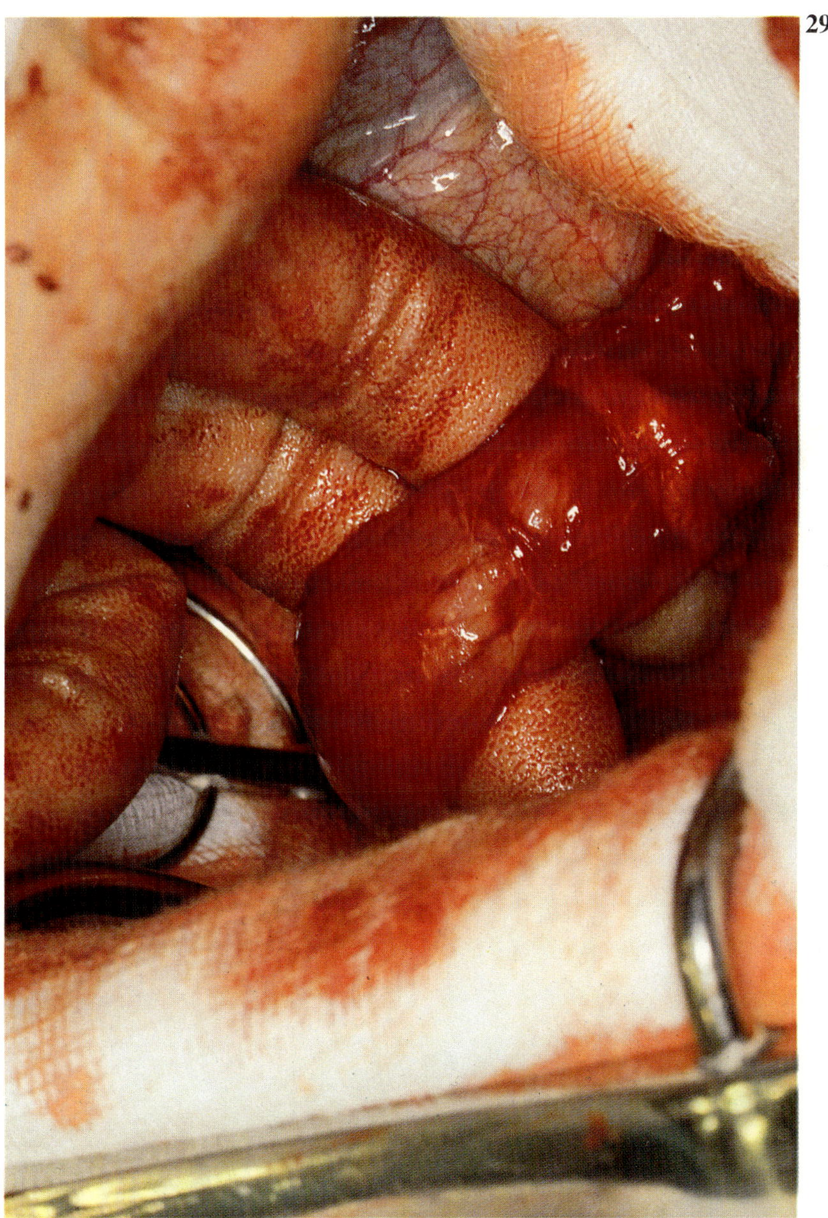

29

30 Placing the sling. A rubber catheter or a piece of tape is then grasped between the opened fingers and drawn back through, behind the oesophagus, and the free ends fastened with a clip in order to act as a sling for the oesophagus. The vagal nerves (anterior and posterior) are easily seen and palpated, and are usually included in the sling.

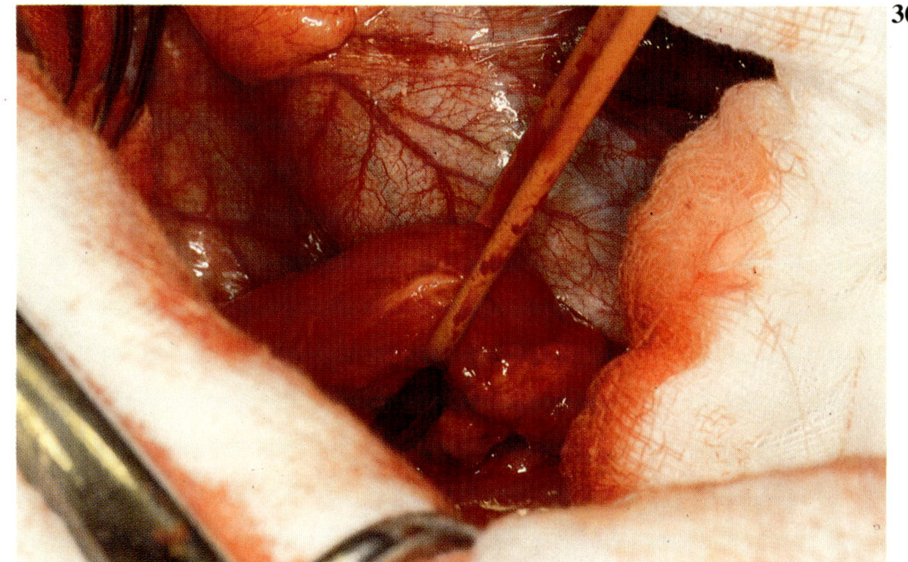

30

31 Gaining oesophageal length. The oesophagus is gradually freed from the surrounding structures by sharp dissection up to the root of the lung after coagulating or tying the small vessels which supply the oesophagus from the aorta. Good haemostasis is essential.

CAUTION: This can be a difficult and very vascular dissection in those patients with much reflux and perioesophagitis.

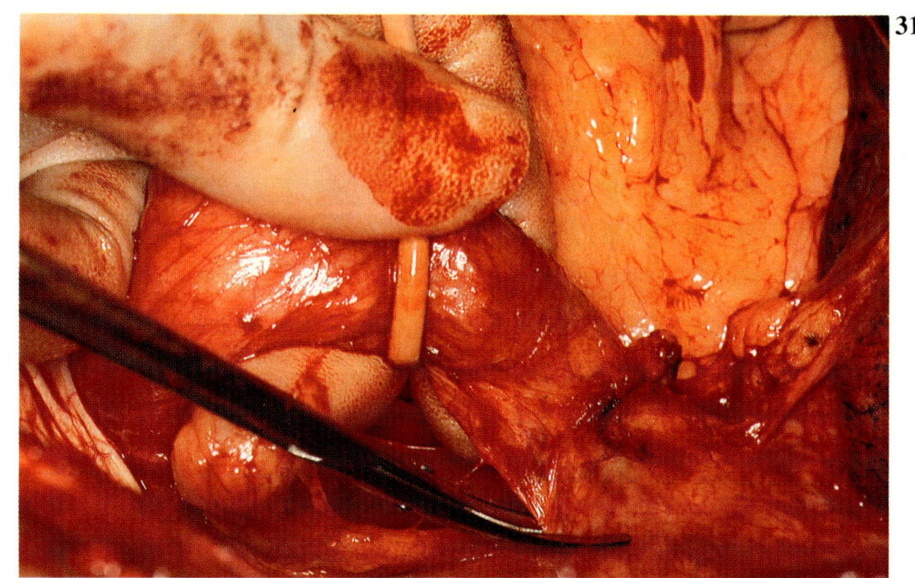

31

32 Continuing the dissection. The dissection is continued distally as far as the oesophageal hiatus.

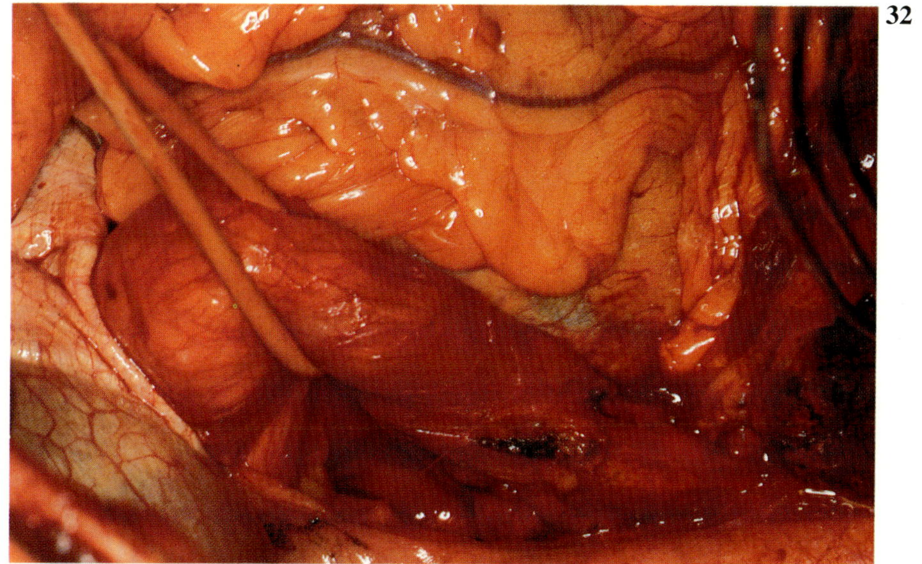
32

33 Identifying the hernial sac. The sac of the hiatal hernia is demonstrated near the hiatus. In this illustration a small hernia is present.

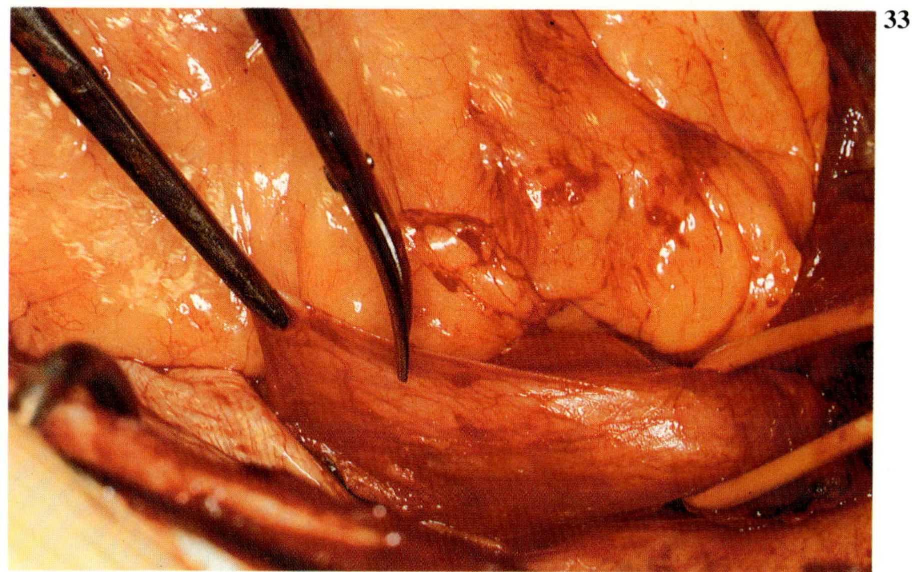
33

34 Opening the sac. The sac is entered near the hiatus and the fundus of the stomach comes into view.

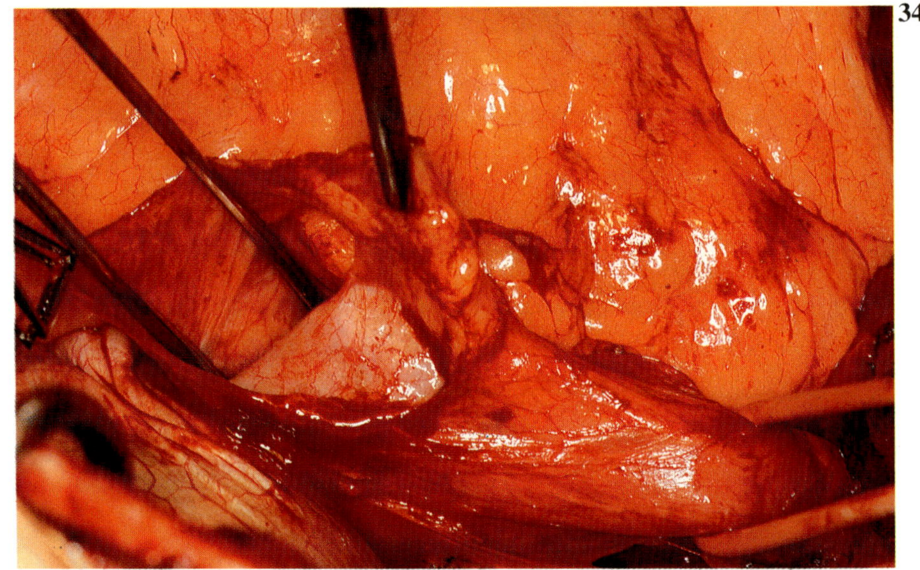

34

35 Removal of sac. In this illustration a much larger hernia is present and this makes the next stage of the dissection easier. All of the fatty tissue and the peritoneal tissue in the wall of the sac must be removed so that the edges of the hiatus are clearly delineated. The lower end of the oesophagus is easily seen at its junction with the stomach.

CAUTION: Removing the pad of fat from the gastrooesophageal junction is always a vascular part of the operation and careful attention must be paid to haemostasis.

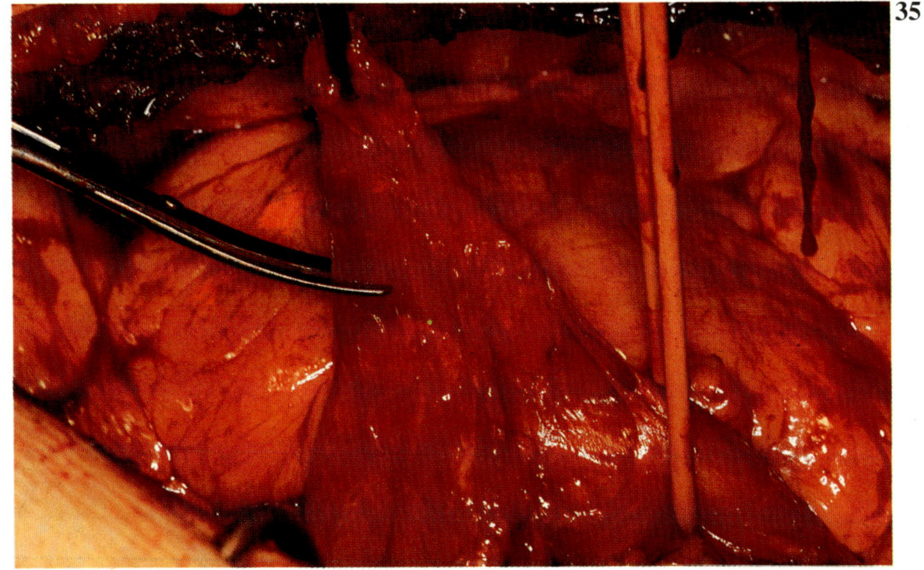

35

36 Exposure of crus. In this illustration the edges of the right crus of the diaphragm have been dissected free of peritoneum and all fatty tissue. The edges of the crus are held in tissue forceps in order to demonstrate the crus. The dissection of the crus must proceed as far back as its origin on each side. This complete delineation of the edges of the hiatus is necessary in order to place, with precision, the stitches for the repair.

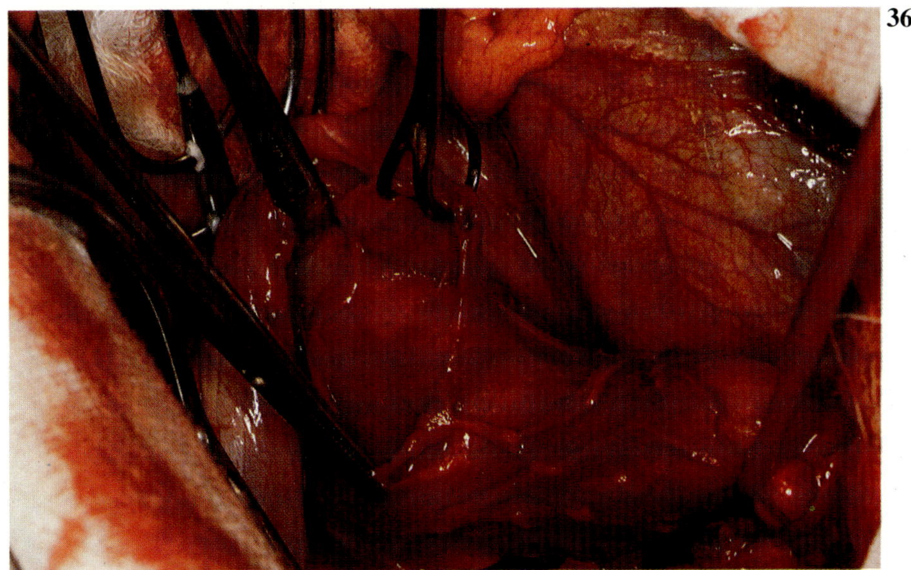
36

37 Anatomy of the repair. The anatomy is displayed prior to beginning the repair. A retractor is used to demonstrate the edge of the hiatus, the stomach fundus has been dislocated into the chest and the oesophagus is seen in the rubber sling. The repair of the crus can now begin.

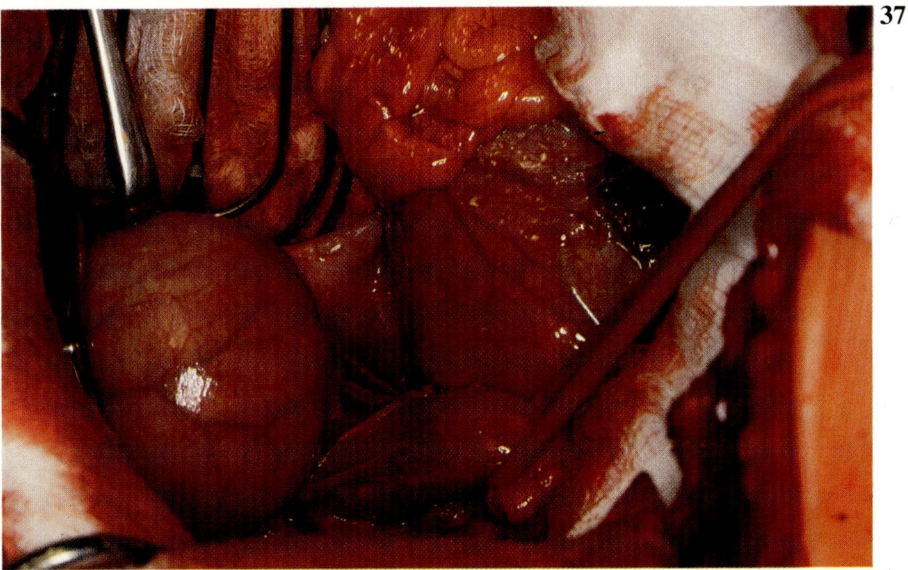
37

38 Suturing the crus. The stomach is dislocated back through the hiatus, and tissue forceps are used to demonstrate the right edge of the crus. Throughout the repair nonabsorbable suture material is used. The author's preference is for Nurolon, threaded or mounted on a round-bodied needle.

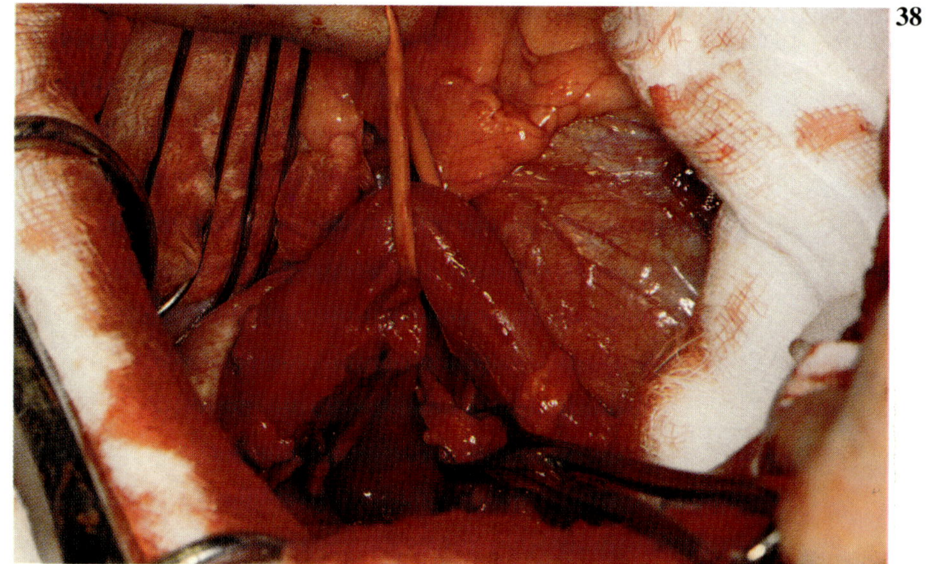

38

39 The first suture. The placing of the first stitch. A No. 1 gauge Nurolon is used for this part of the repair. The stitch has been passed through the right margin of the crus near its origin. The needle is then repositioned prior to passing the stitch through the left margin of the crus as far posteriorly as possible.

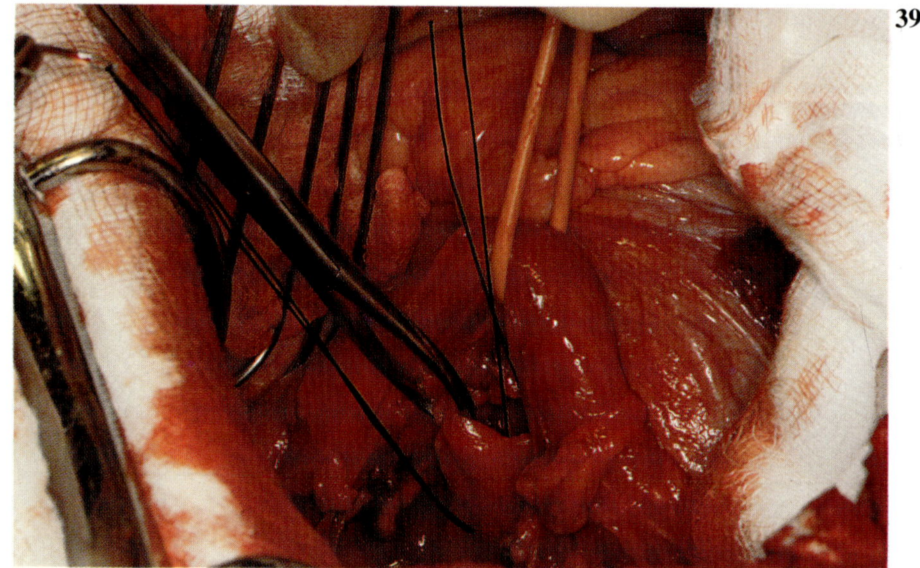

39

40

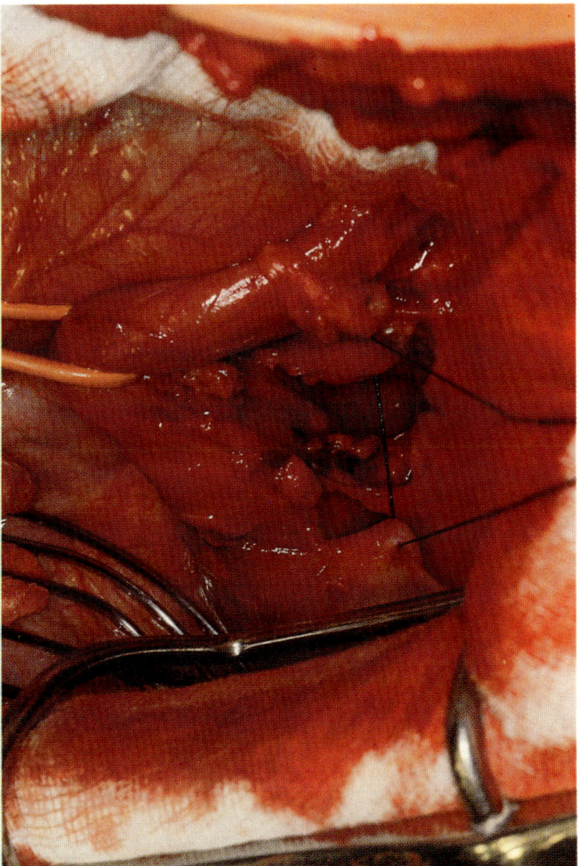

41

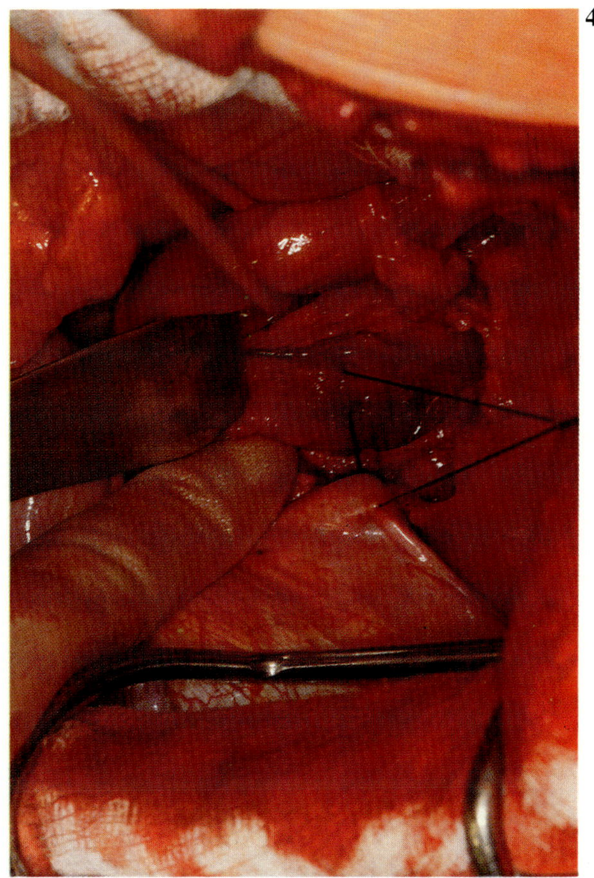

40 The completed first suture. The insertion of the first suture through the muscle fibres of the right crus has been completed. It is helpful while inserting this stich for the assistant to retract the crus so that the surgeon has a firm band of muscle both to palpate and to see. The suture is not tied at this stage of the operation but is loosely held in a clip.

41 Use of retractor. A copper retractor, which can be bent into a convenient shape, is useful for holding the stomach and oesophagus forward so that the sutures in the crus can be placed accurately and the edges of the crus can be declared. The use of this retractor and its value in exposure can easily be seen here. The index finger is inserted into the hiatus at this stage to determine whether or not further sutures are required to narrow the hiatus.

42

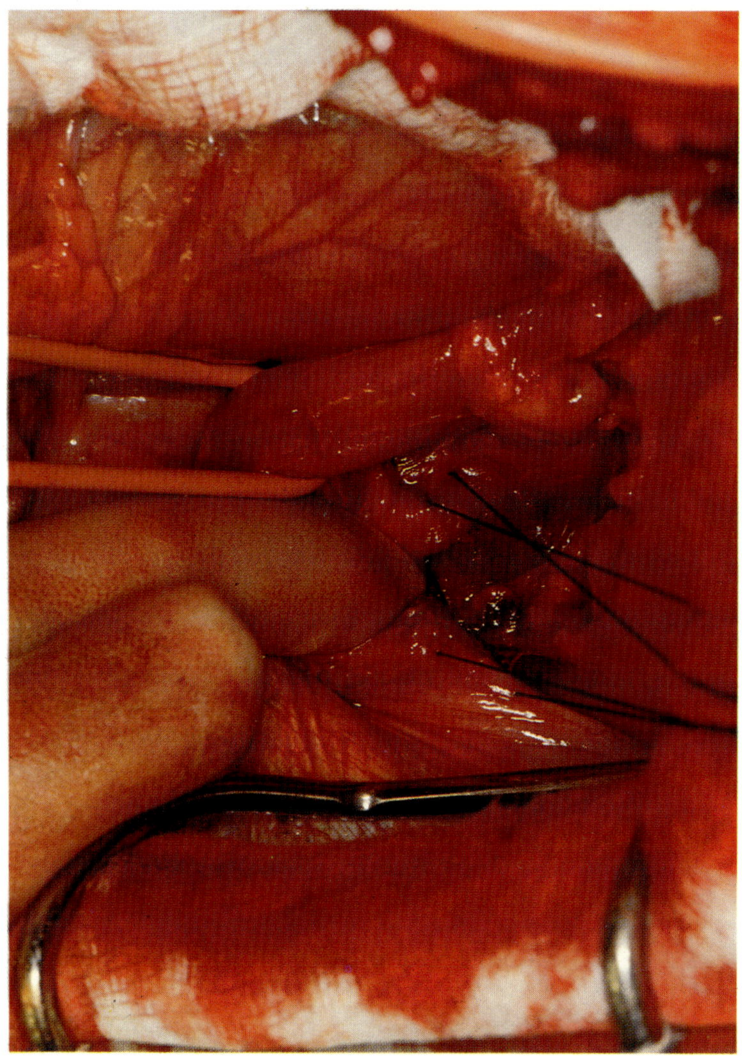

42 Assessment of size of hiatus. Judgement is required to decide how many sutures to insert but it is better to insert too many at this stage. Later in the operation when these sutures are tied it is easy to remove the most anterior one if the hiatal repair is too tight, but it is almost impossible to insert an additional suture if the repair is too slack. The ideal is to allow just enough room for the tip of the index finger to lie between the sutured crus and the posterior surface of the oesophagus. This illustration demonstrates this way of assessing the need for sutures.

43 Large defects. Sometimes, especially with very large defects, it is easier to start suturing from the front backwards and as is shown here the first stitch is placed with the index finger being used to determine the size of the hiatus as the ends of the suture are pulled. This view also shows the posterior edges of the defect in the right crus and demonstrates that many sutures will be required to close this large defect.

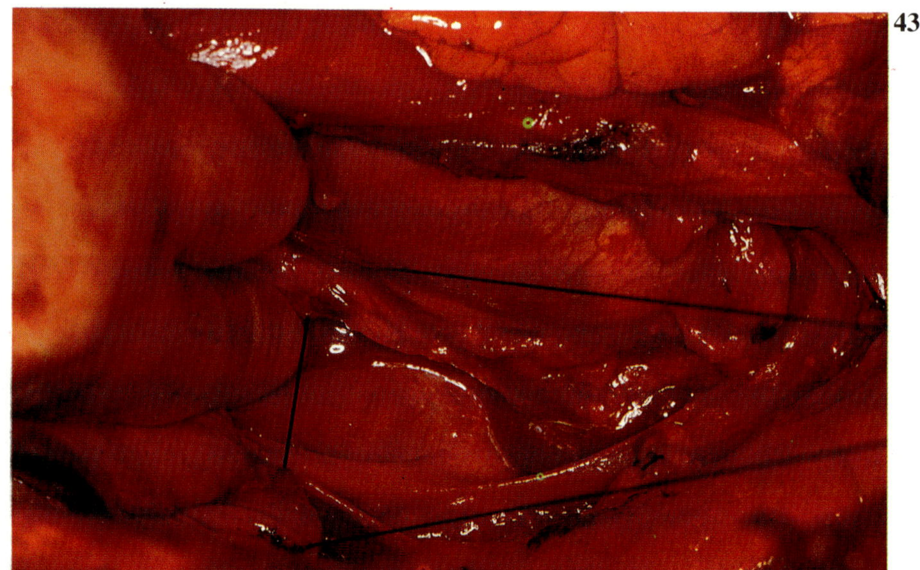

43

44 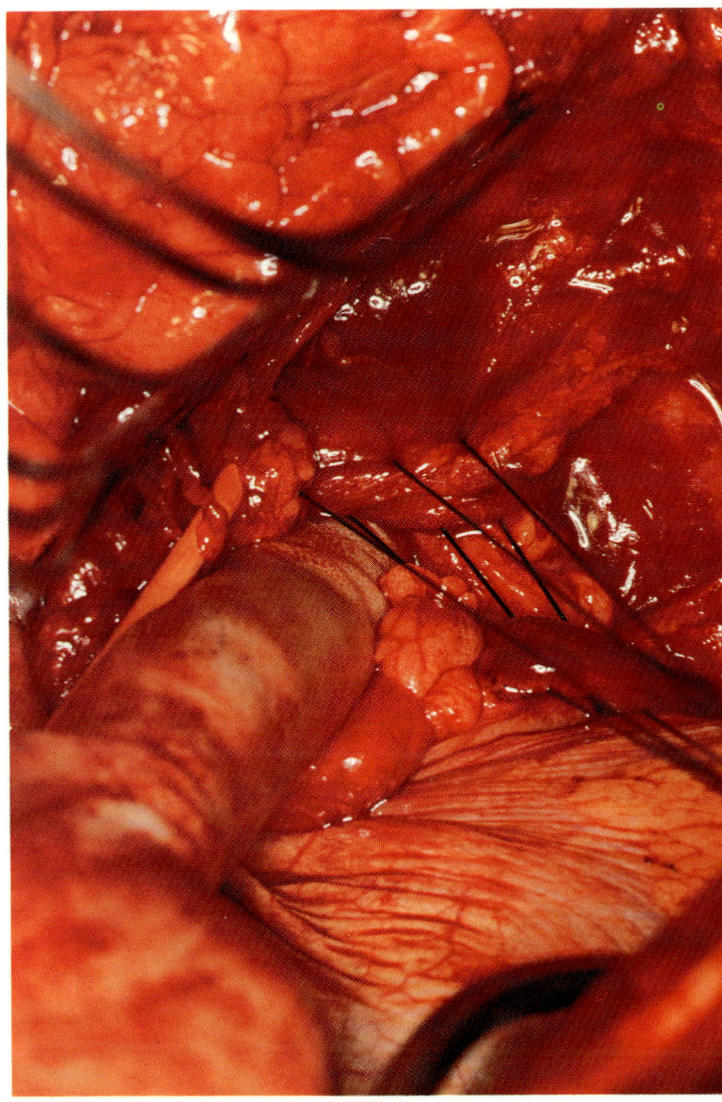

44 Suturing a large defect. Here three sutures have been inserted but another two or three will be required posteriorly.

CAUTION: Remember these sutures are not tied at this point but are held in clips to be tied as the final part of the repair. Indeed it is advisable to slacken off these crural sutures after insertion as it makes the next stage of the repair easier

45 The anatomical aim. The next stage of the operation involves recreating a lower end of oesophagus which is intraabdominal and which has a cuff of gastric fundus wrapped round part of the circumference of the oesophagus. If enough oesophagus has been mobilised as described above in **19-32** it may be possible to have 3-5 cm of oesophagus below the diaphragm. Of course this may be difficult in patients with long standing oesophagitis and the associated shortening of the oesophagus. The first step in this part of the operation consists of bringing the stomach back into the chest through the hiatus.

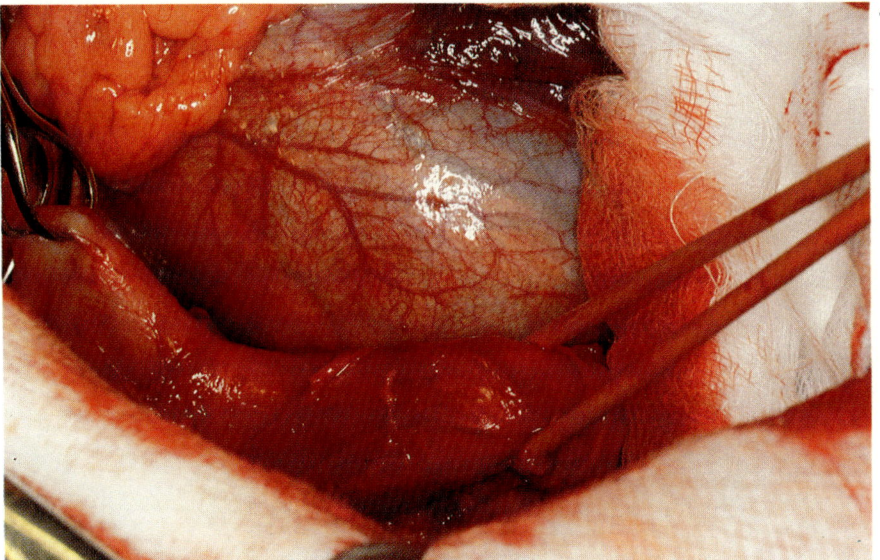 45

46

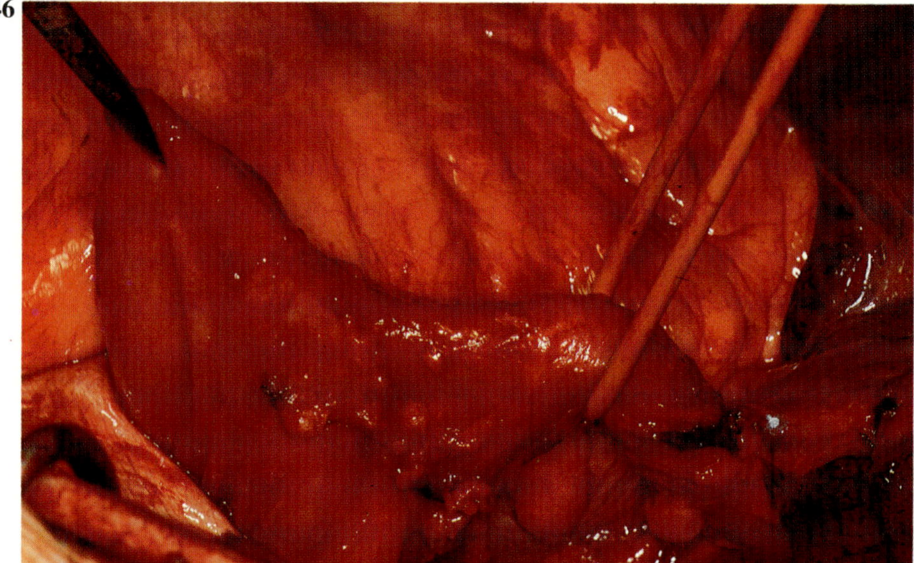

47

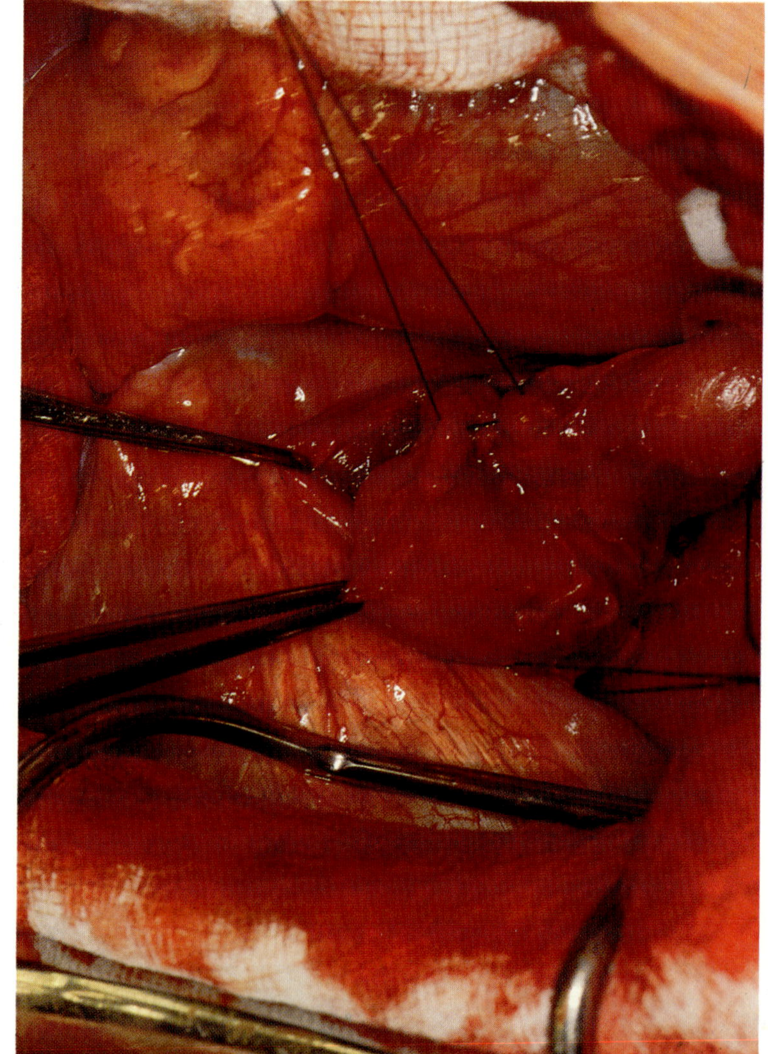

46 If the mobilisation has been carried out properly a considerable portion of the upper end of the stomach can be brought through the hiatus. This makes the subsequent suturing fairly easy.

47 The first layer. This layer of sutures serves to begin turning a cuff of gastric fundus so that it lies along the left side of the lower end of the oesophagus for a length of 1.5-2 cm. This illustration shows the first of these stitches being placed as far medially as possible. The stitch picks up the muscle of the lower end of the oesophagus about 1.5-2 cm above the oesophagogastric junction and then a seromuscular bite of the fundus of the stomach about the same distance below the gastrooesophageal junction. The suture is tied. The suture material used is 2/0 Nurolon on a round-bodied needle.

48

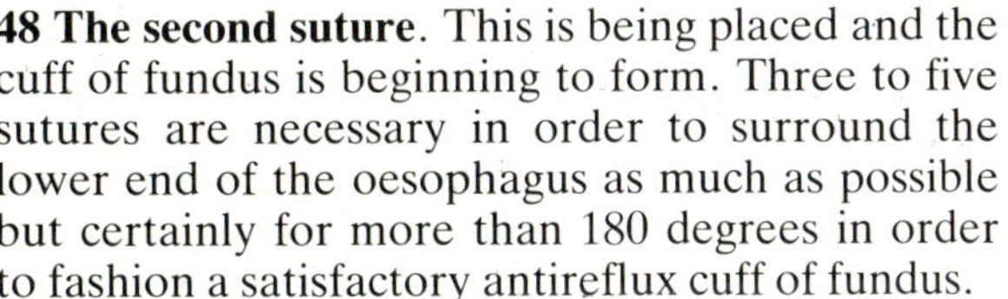

48 The second suture. This is being placed and the cuff of fundus is beginning to form. Three to five sutures are necessary in order to surround the lower end of the oesophagus as much as possible but certainly for more than 180 degrees in order to fashion a satisfactory antireflux cuff of fundus.

49

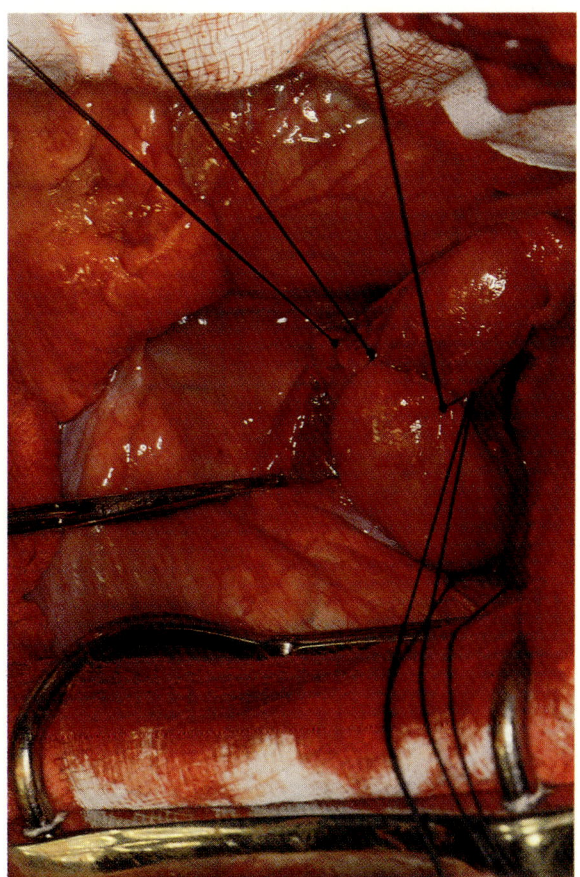

49 First layer complete. Four sutures have been used here and the fundus of the stomach covers the lower part of the oesophagus when these are tied.

50

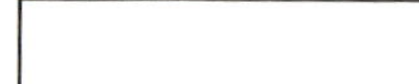

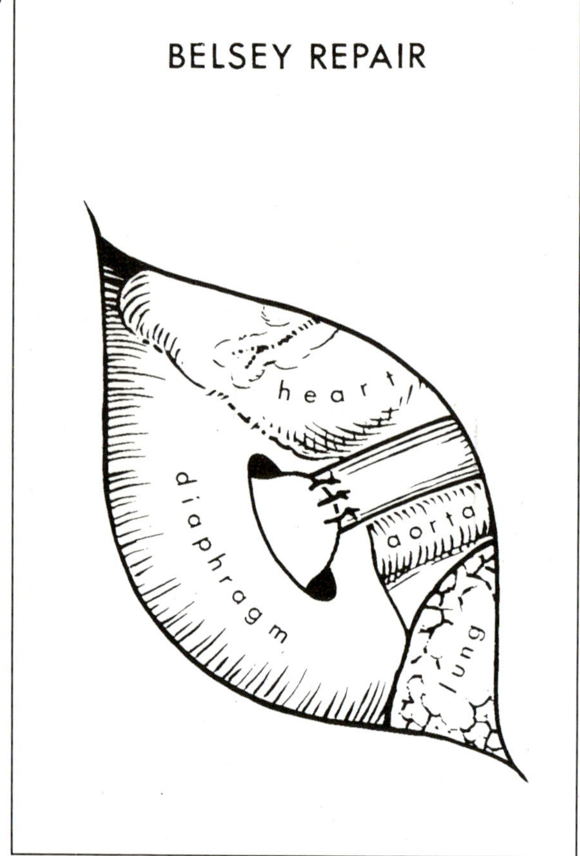

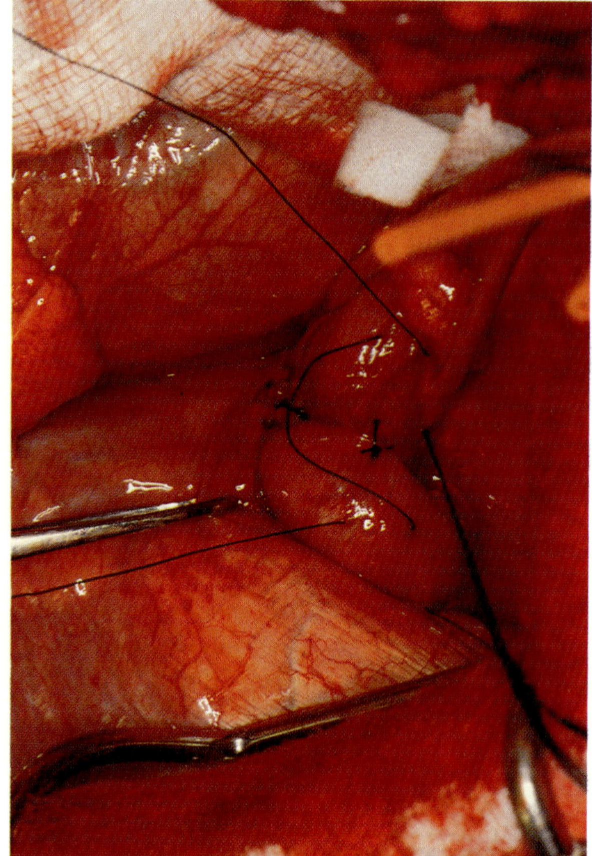

51

50 The first layer of sutures (diagram). In practice, as is shown in **47-49**, the wrap round of the lower end of the oesophagus by the fundus is much greater.

51 The second layer. The second layer of sutures is more difficult to understand and to carry out. Its purpose is to bring more of the gastric fundal cuff over the lower end of oesophagus, to position the lower end of oesophagus with the gastric fundal cuff through the hiatus and to hold the intraabdominal oesophagus in position below the diaphragm. This should all be achieved without tension if the oesophagus has been mobilised enough in a proximal fashion, (see **31**). If the tension is too great then the oesophagus will have to be mobilised more proximally by reflecting the root of the lung forwards and mobilising more of the oesophagus from its bed.

52

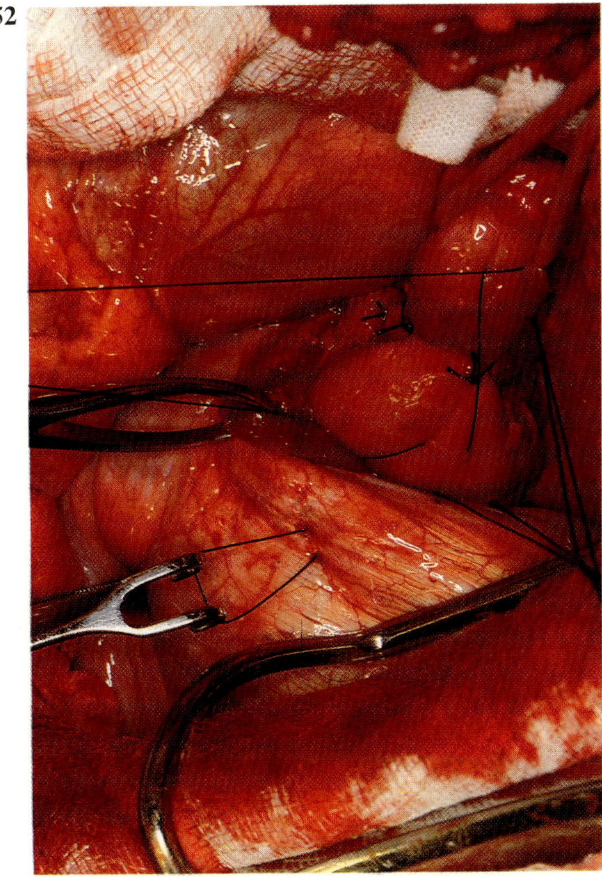

53

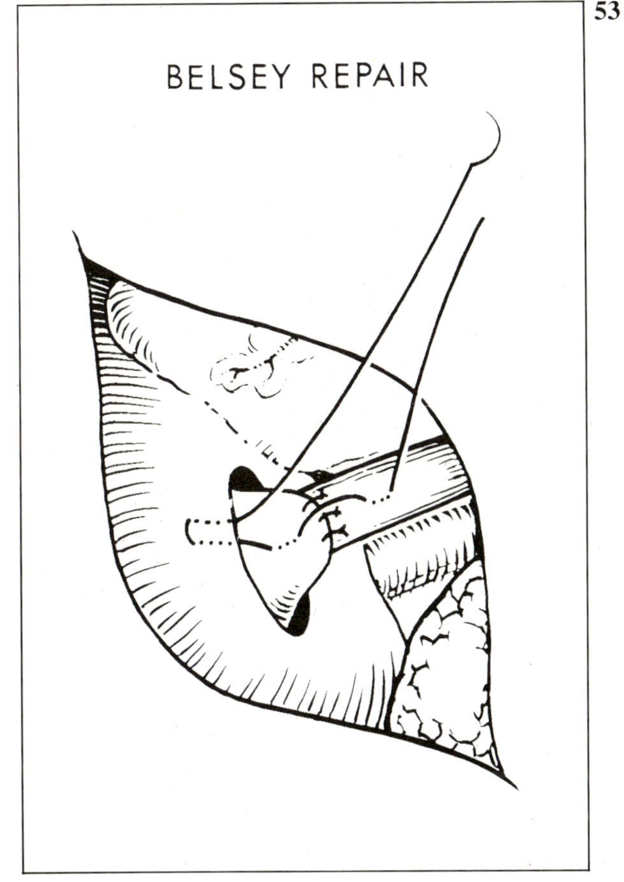

52 The suture is continued. The needle is passed through the diaphragm from within the hiatus and then back through, as shown, to complete each suture. This is demonstrated in the figure by the double hook which is holding the loop which passes through the diaphragm. The edge of the hiatus is shown by the tissue forceps. Although only one suture is shown in the illustration for clarity, three or four sutures are used to complete the second layer which covers more than 180 degrees of the circumference of the lower end of the oesophagus.
Some surgeons begin and end the stitch at the diaphragm.

53 A drawing of the suture. The steps in performing the suture described in 51 and 52 are shown in this drawing.

CAUTION: The needle being passed through the hiatus and through the diaphragm is in danger of causing bleeding from the vessels on the undersurface of the diaphragm or from damage to the splenic capsule. Indeed damage can be caused without the operator being aware of it because the bleeding is concealed by the diaphragm. This can be avoided by using a similar technique to that shown in the next figure.

54

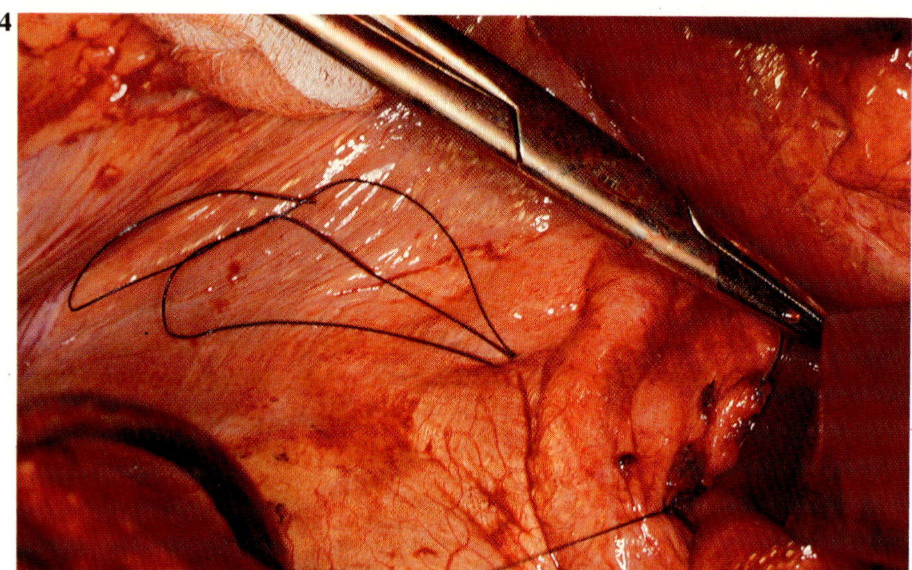

55

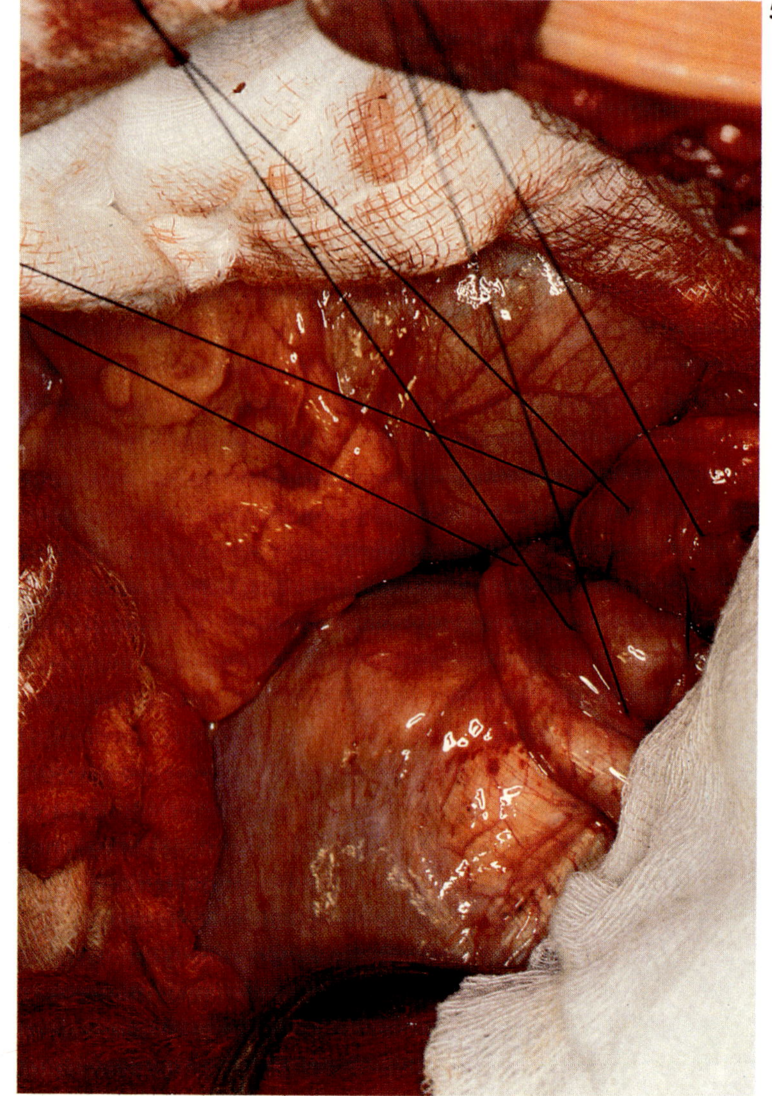

54 The retractor. The adjacent structures are protected by using a copper malleable retractor when passing the needle through the diaphragm as described in **52**. The presence of the retractor also enables bleeding from under the diaphragm to be seen readily, as it accumulates on the surface of the retractor.

55 Second layer complete. The second layer has been completed and the stiches are about to be tied. There is little tension and the gastric fundus and lower end of oesophagus are about to disappear through the hiatus.

CAUTION: If the tension is too great then these sutures will cut out, especially from the oesophagus, when an attempt is made to tie them. In some patients, where the tissue is particularly friable, the use of little Teflon patches to reinforce the poor tissue of oesophagus or stomach has been suggested by Belsey but the author has not found these useful. He prefers, where it can be achieved, to have as little tension as possible in order to avoid the sutures cutting out.

56 Closure of the hiatus. The second layer of sutures has been tied and the lower end of oesophagus and the gastric fundus are now held below the diaphragm in the normal anatomical position.

Attention is now turned to the sutures which were placed in the right crus of the diaphragm as described in **38-44**. Starting with the most posterior, each suture is tied firmly and the oesophageal hiatus is narrowed. The next suture is now approximated and this process continues anteriorly until all the sutures have been tied. When completed the hiatus should just allow the insertion of the tip of the index finger between the posterior surface of the oesophagus and the last suture tied. When the surgeon has decided that the oesophageal hiatus has been narrowed enough then the remaining sutures are not tied, but removed.

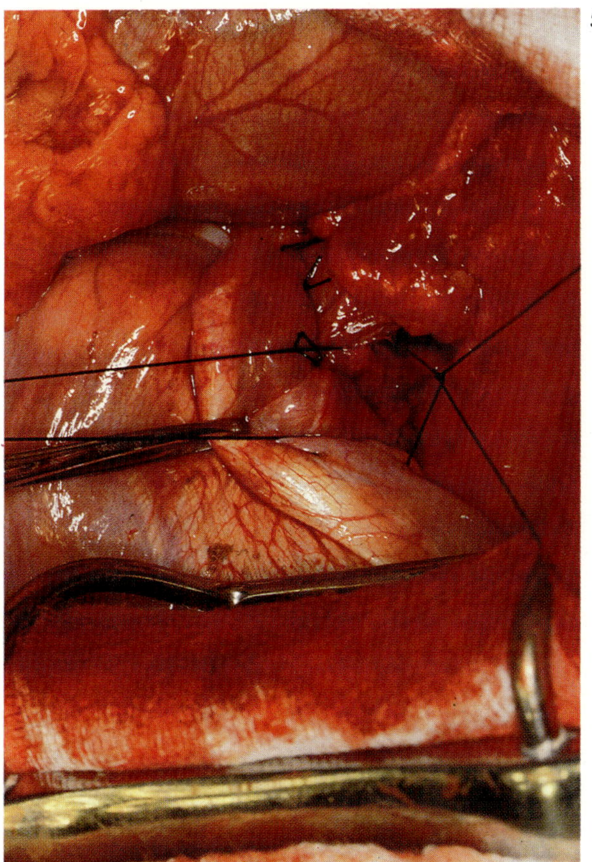

56

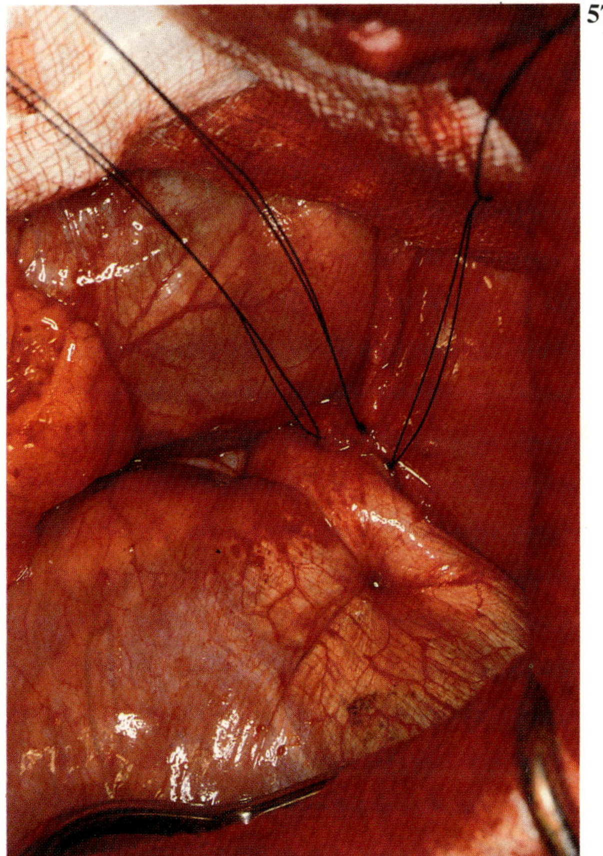

57

57 Final sutures. The author inserts a few final sutures to close off the adjacent edge of the hiatus to the oesophagus. The suture material used is 3/0 Nurolon.

58

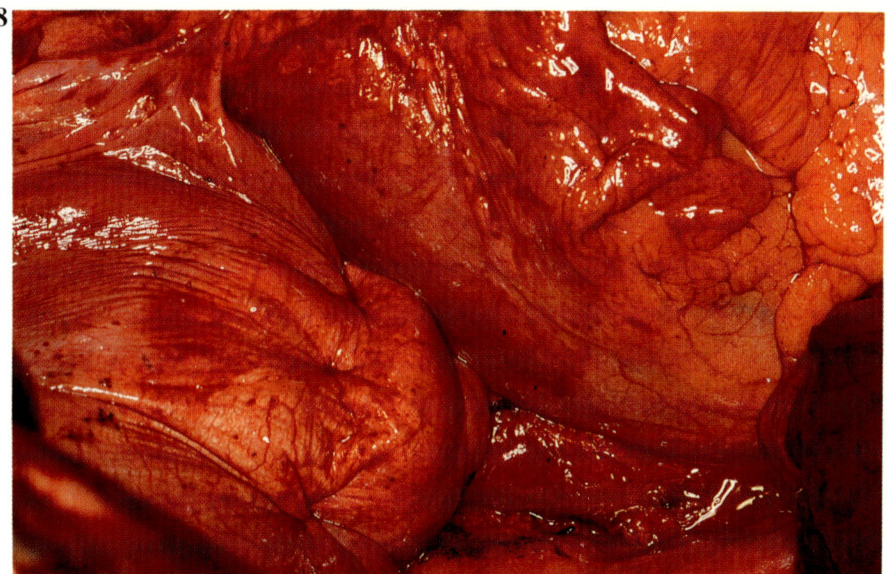

58 Replacing the oesophagus. The oesophagus is now replaced in its bed in the mediastinum.

CAUTION: Haemostasis should be as complete as possible before the operator begins to close the thoracotomy incision

59

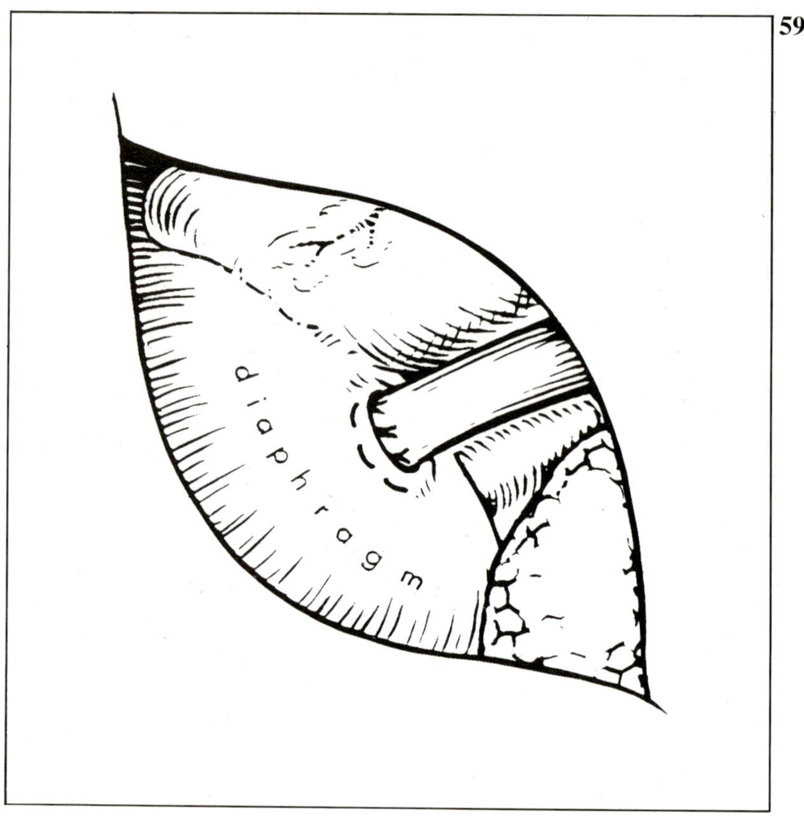

59 Belsey repair. The completed operation (diagram).

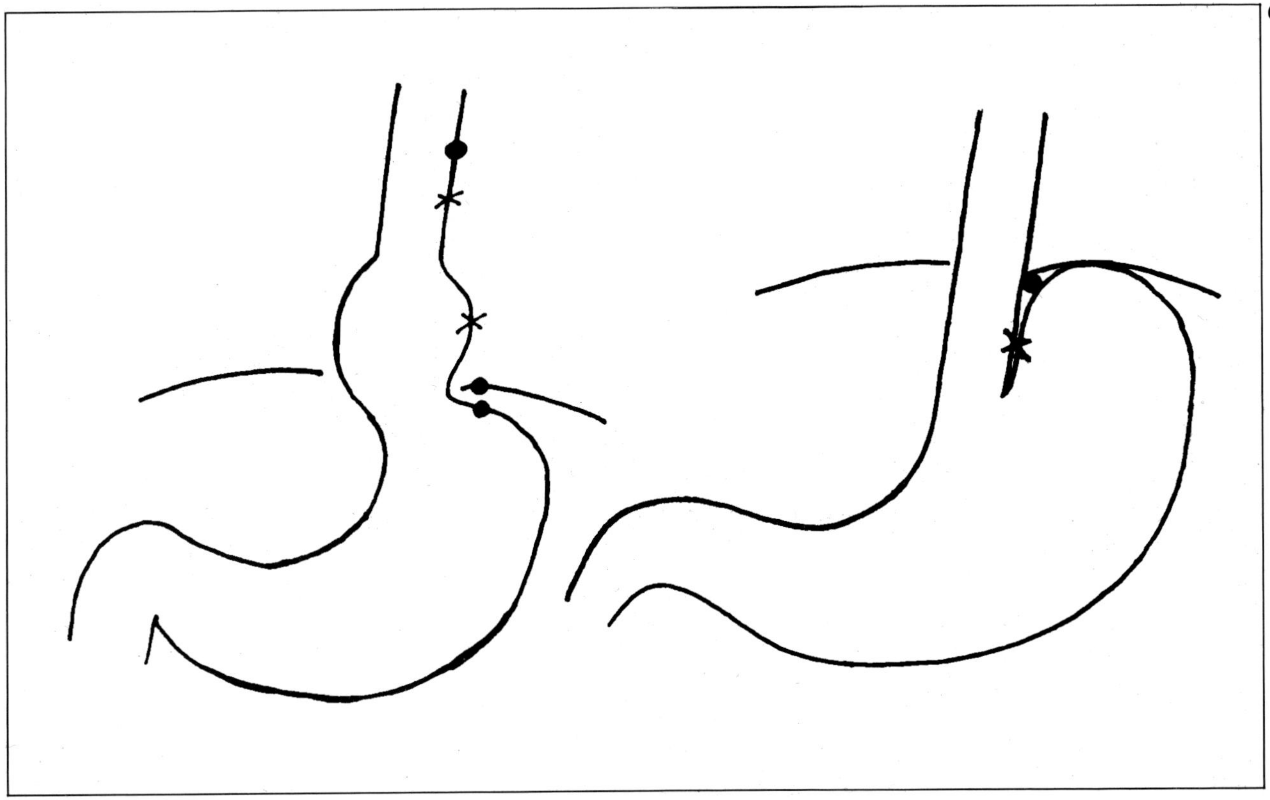

60 Summary of steps in repair. These line drawings summarise the steps in the repair. The first layer sutures together the sites marked with crosses (×) in the drawing on the left. The second layer of sutures approximates those points marked with circles (•) on the left. The drawing on the right shows the effect of approximating the layers as described. The lower end of the oesophagus is covered by a cuff of gastric fundus, the acute angle between lower end of oesophagus and gastric fundus is restored, the oblique angle of entry of the oesophagus into the stomach is re-established and finally the lower oesophagus becomes intra-abdominal and is retained below the diaphragm. As a result the normal anatomical situation is restored–the condition most suitable for the control of reflux. The concept of the Belsy repair has been fulfilled.

Closure of thoracotomy

61

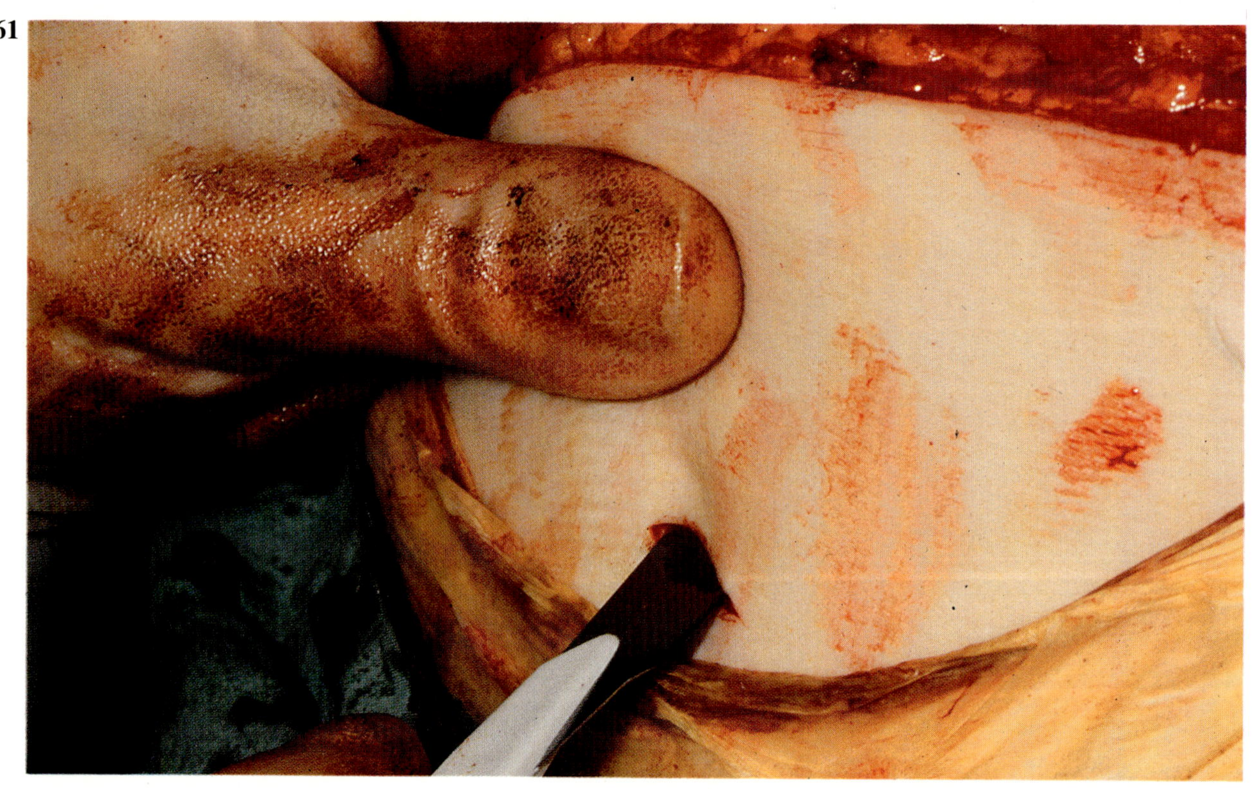

61 Siting of chest drain incision. The retractor is removed from the thoracotomy wound and the protective plastic film, if used, is peeled off the edges of the incision. The hand is placed into the left chest at the lower edge of the wound and a position is selected in the mid axillary line just above the insertion of the diaphragm to the lateral wall of the chest for the chest drain to come through.

A small incision is made with the tip of a scalpel just above a rib and this incision is deepened until the scalpel can just be felt coming through at the point selected by the left hand. The deepening of the incision through the parietal pleura can be performed using a heavy pair of haemostatic forceps through the skin incision if the operator prefers.

CAUTION: The positioning of the thoracic drain is very important as it must lie where it cannot be blocked by the weight of the patient lying on it. It is for this reason that the author prefers the midaxillary line.

62 Pleural drain. The author uses a size 24 Mallinckrodt catheter for drainage of the pleural cavity. Obviously the size of the catheter is related to the size of the patient and on many occasions a smaller drain can be used but it is important to use as big a catheter as possible to enable free drainage of blood and to prevent blockage when clot is present. Many other manufacturers produce equally suitable chest drains and the operator should use the one he prefers, providing the walls of the drain are thick enough and the drain incision is adequate enough to prevent collapse of the drain at the point at which it comes through the chest wall.

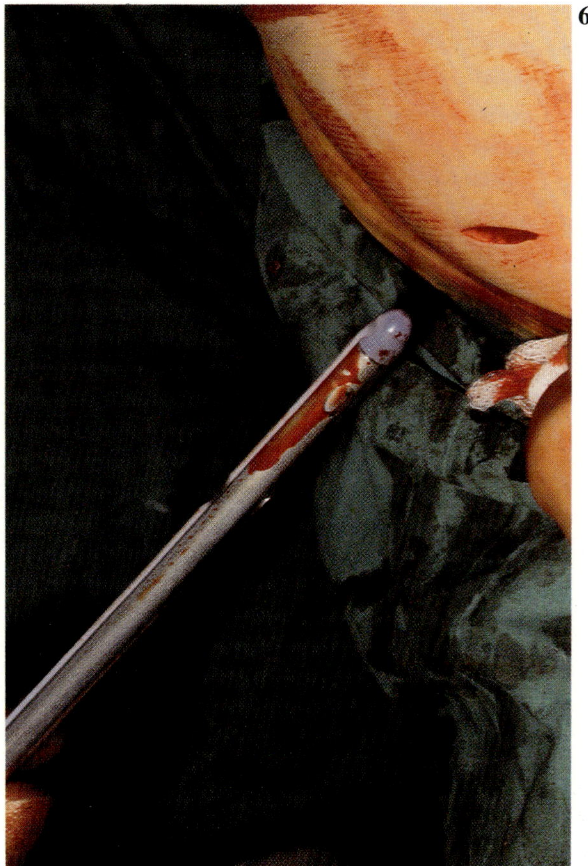

62

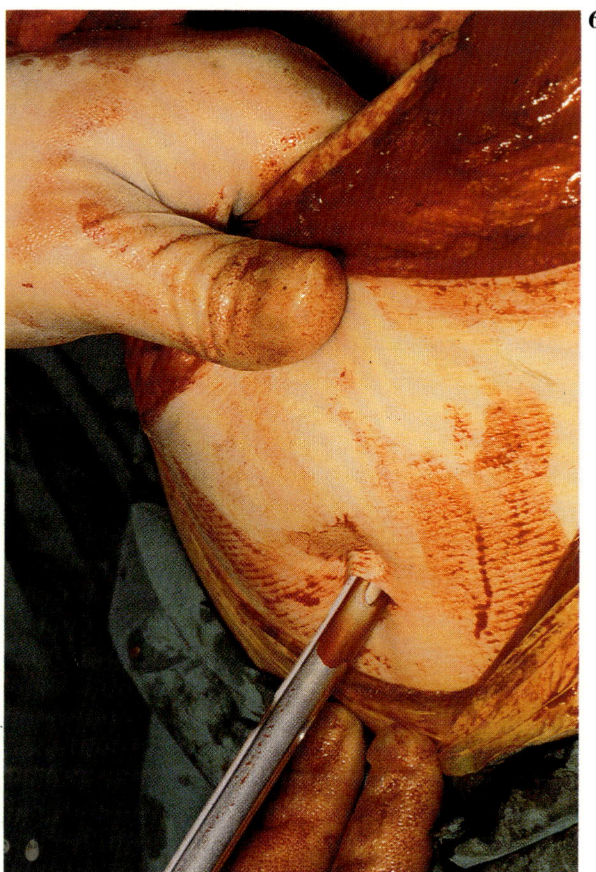

63

63 Insertion of drain. The catheter, complete with its introducer, is passed through the small incision in the chest wall and the obturator is removed. The tip of the drain is placed in the paravertebral gutter at the level of the upper limit of the mediastinal dissection.

64 Fixation of catheter. A stitch is used to fix the drain at the point at which it enters the chest wall. Many surgeons also place a purse string suture, which is left untied, round the drain so that it can be used to close the small chest wall incision when the catheter is removed.

The chest drain is not connected to the drainage apparatus at this point in the operation. The author prefers to leave this until after the ribs have been prepared for approximation and the lung has been inflated.

64

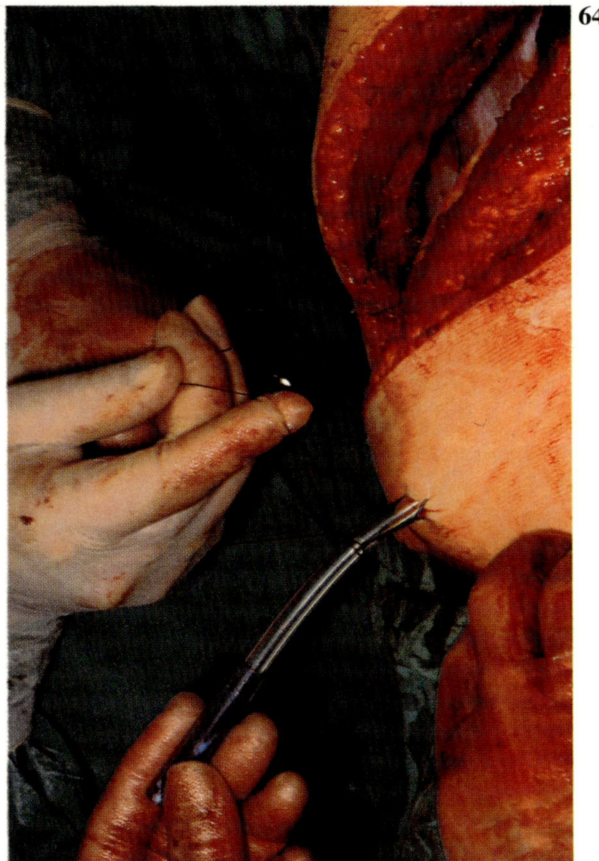

65

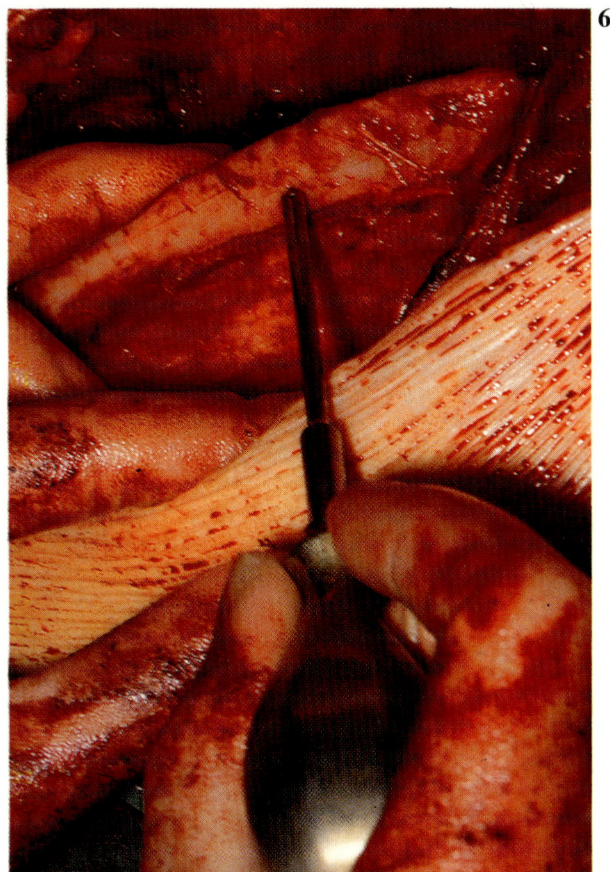

65 Use of bone awl. The bone awl should have an eye big enough to accept a suitable suture for the rib stitch. Monofilament nylon is used for this purpose but some surgeons use steel and others chromic catgut. In the author's opinion it is essential to fix the ribs in order to diminish postoperative chest pain. A bone awl is used so that a circumferential suture does not crush the intercostal nerve as it lies in the subcostal groove.

66

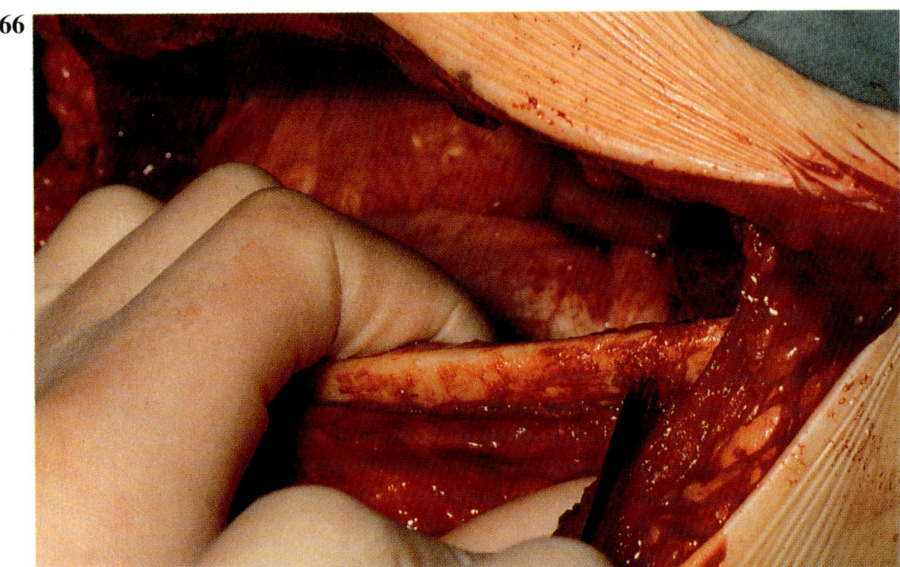

67

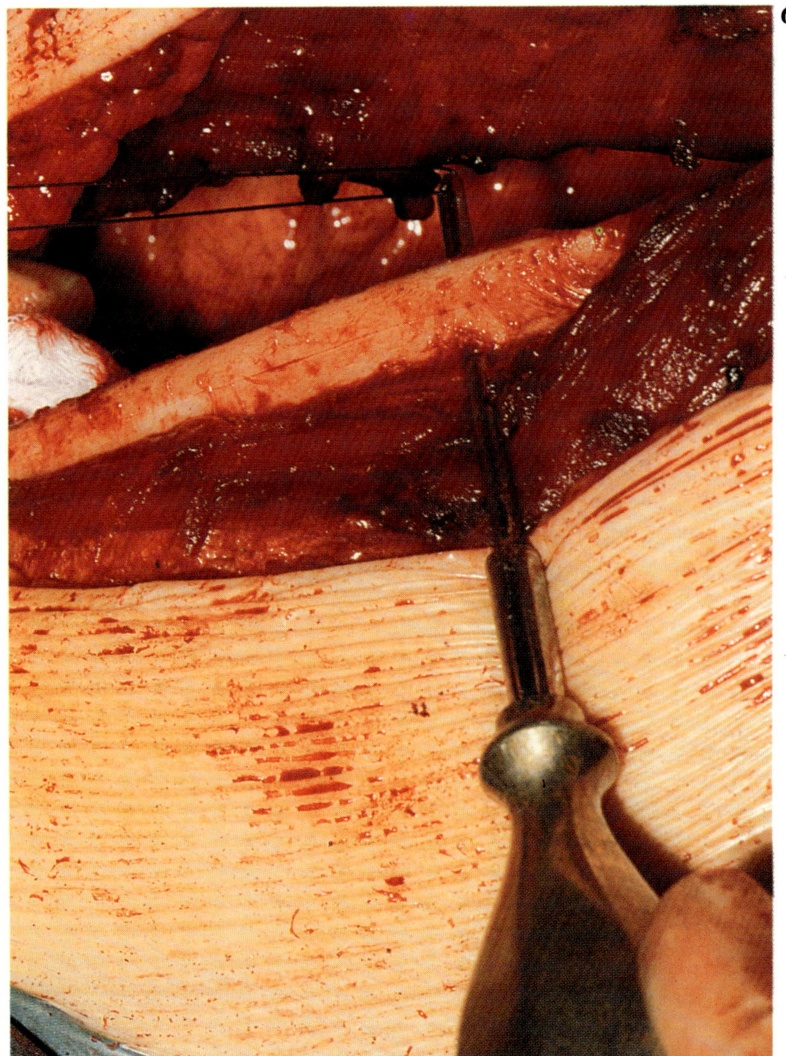

66 Piercing the rib. The bone awl is placed midway between the superior and inferior borders of the lower rib in the incision and it is rotated to and fro until it penetrates the rib. The point chosen for this penetration is at the junction of the posterior and middle third of the exposed lower rib.

67 Threading the awl. The distal end of the monofilament nylon suture is threaded through the eye of the awl and the awl is then withdrawn from the rib, leaving the suture protruding from the hole in the rib.

68

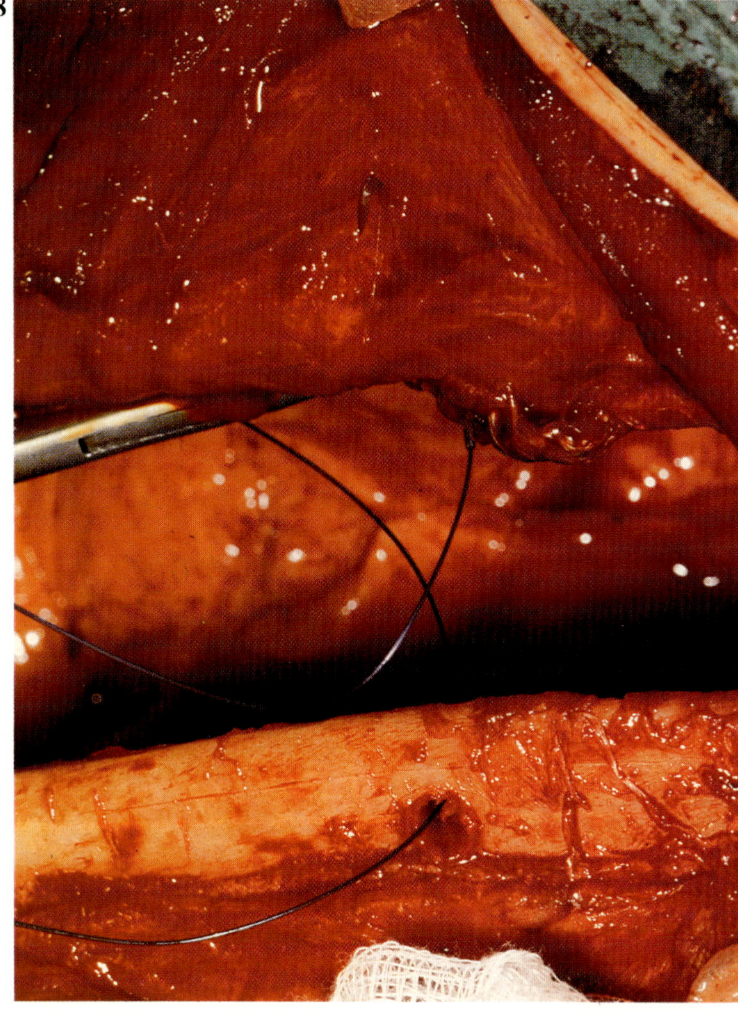

68 Completing the stitch. The needle on the proximal end of the suture is then passed through from within the pleural cavity just above the rib in the upper edge of the incision. A suitable length of suture is selected and then the needle is cut off and the ends of the suture held in a clip. The bone awl can be used on the upper rib as well, rather than having a circumferential stitch round the upper rib.

69 A similar suture is placed at the junction of the middle third and the anterior third of the incision. This suture is also held in a clip, but not tied at this point in the operation.

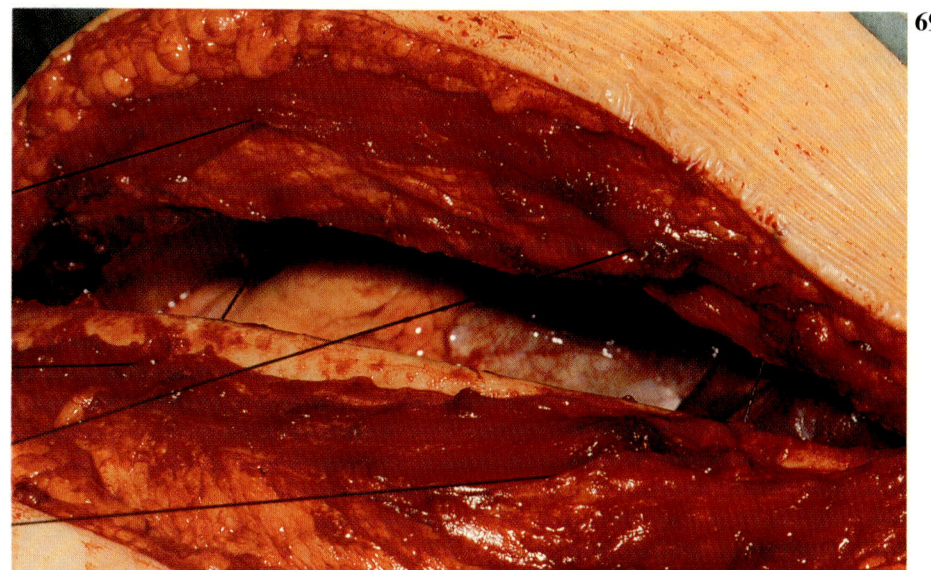

69

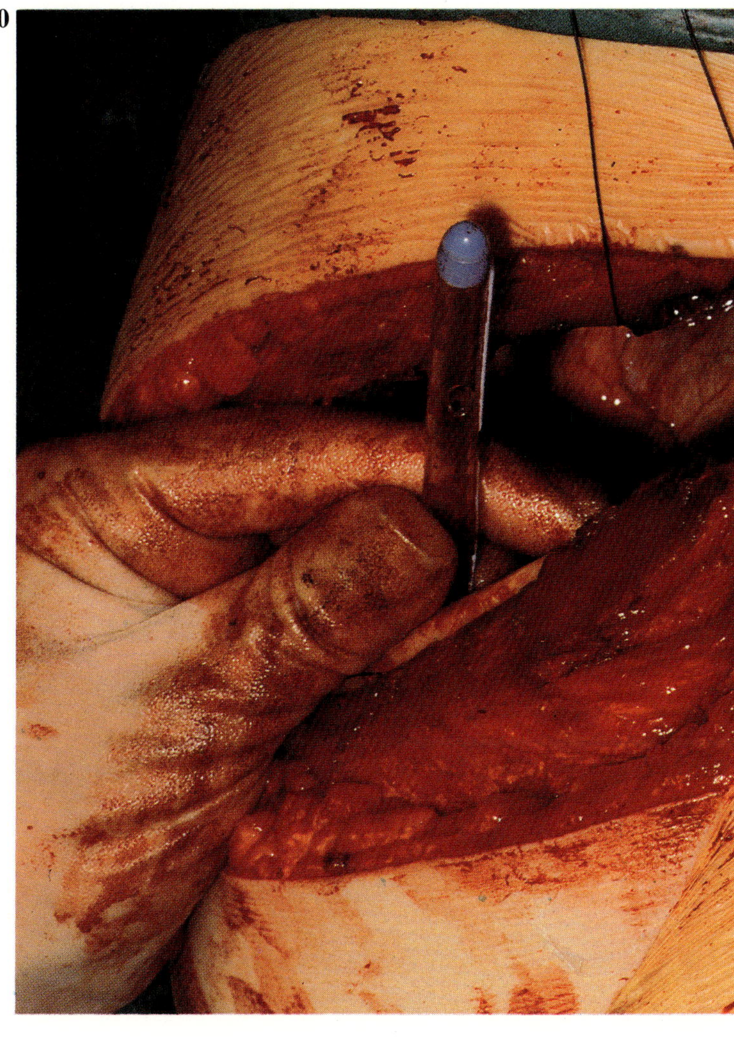

70 Final checks. When it is confirmed that there is no bleeding in the pleural cavity, that any residual blood has been sucked out, that the drain openings are free of clot, the drain is repositioned in the paravertebral gutter as described in **63**.

71 Inflation of lung. The collapsed lung is now inspected for any lacerations or damage and the anaesthetist is asked to inflate the lung.

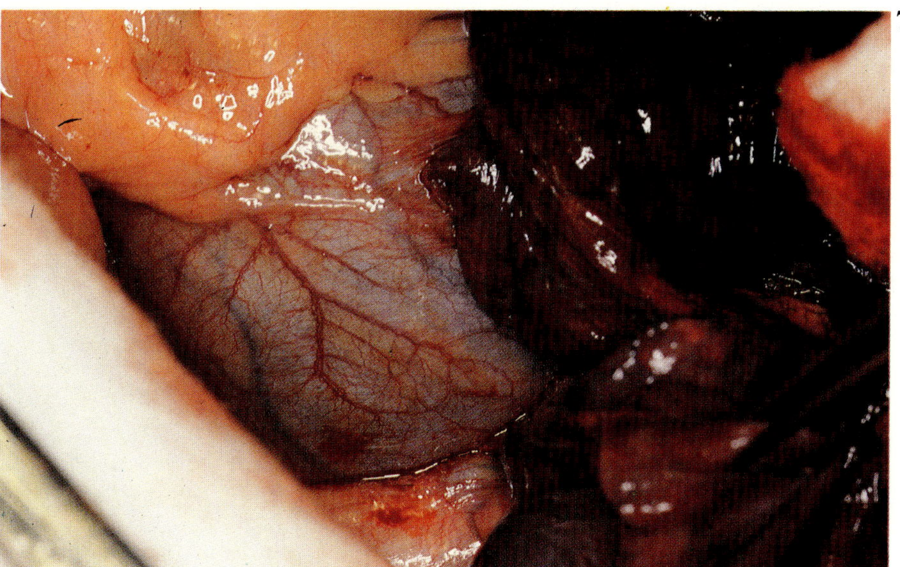

71

72 Areas of collapse. As the lung inflates the surgeon helps by teasing collapsed areas with the fingers to encourage inflation. It is important that the lingula is checked for complete inflation as it may be more reluctant to expand than other parts of the upper lobe. In this photograph the tip of the lingula can be seen inflated while the lower lobe is still collapsed.

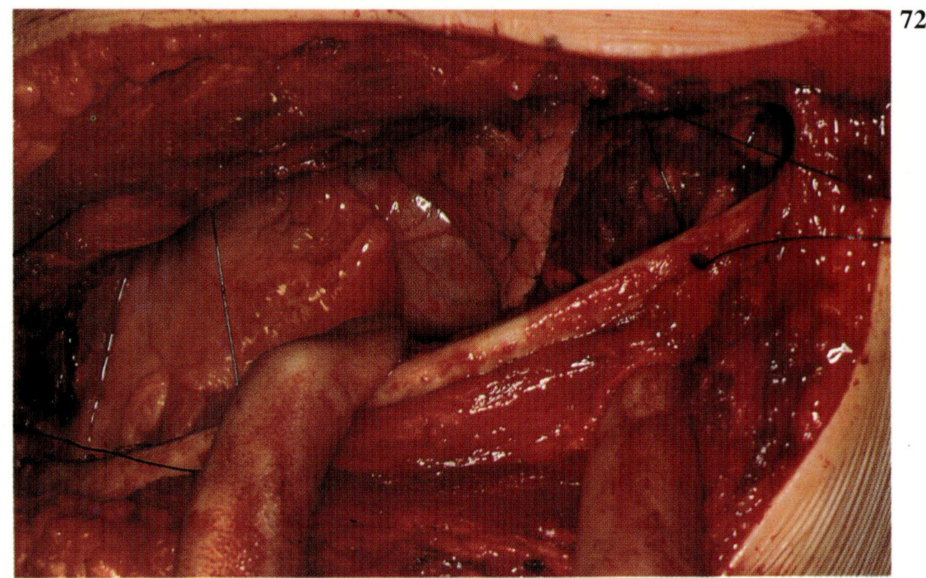
72

73 Checking for inflation. It is important to check along the edges of the lobes to make sure that expansion is complete.

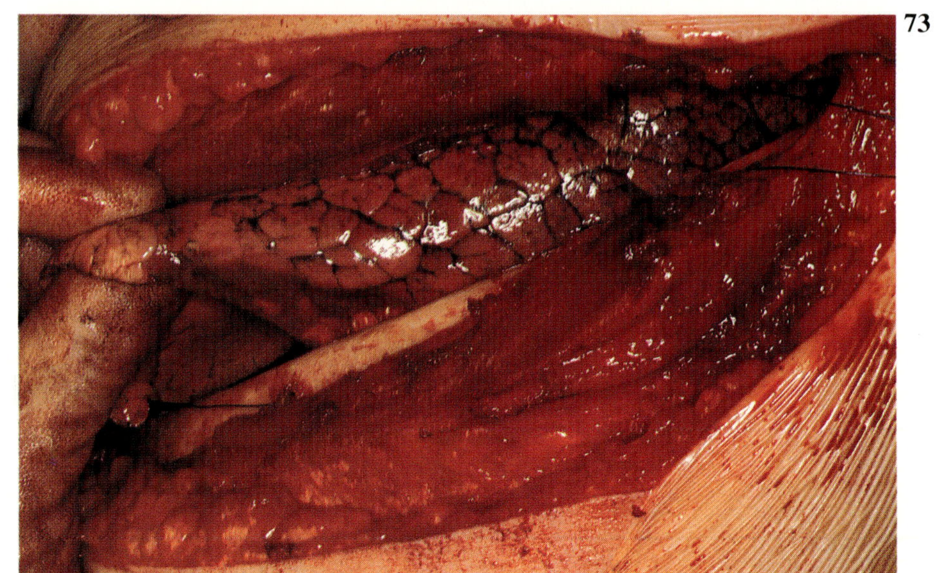
73

74

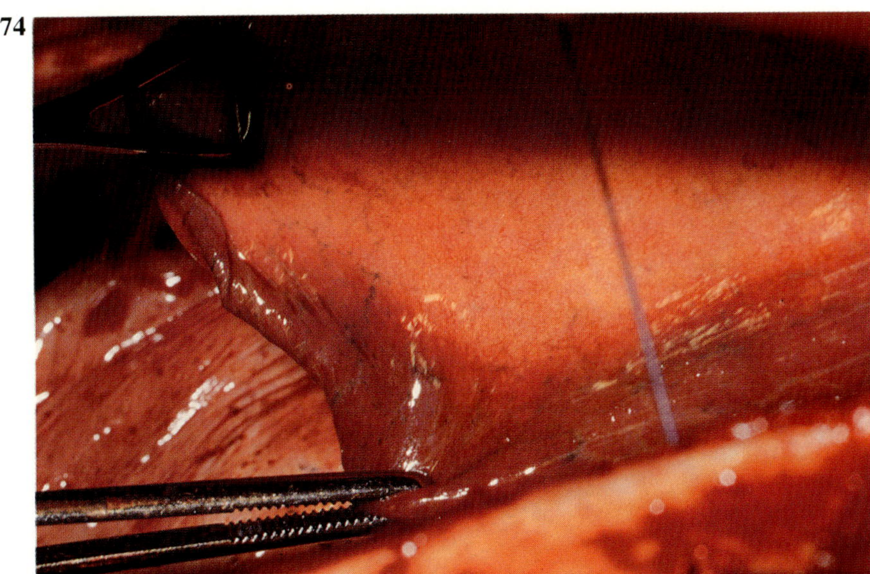

74 Areas of collapse along the edges of the lower lobe.

75

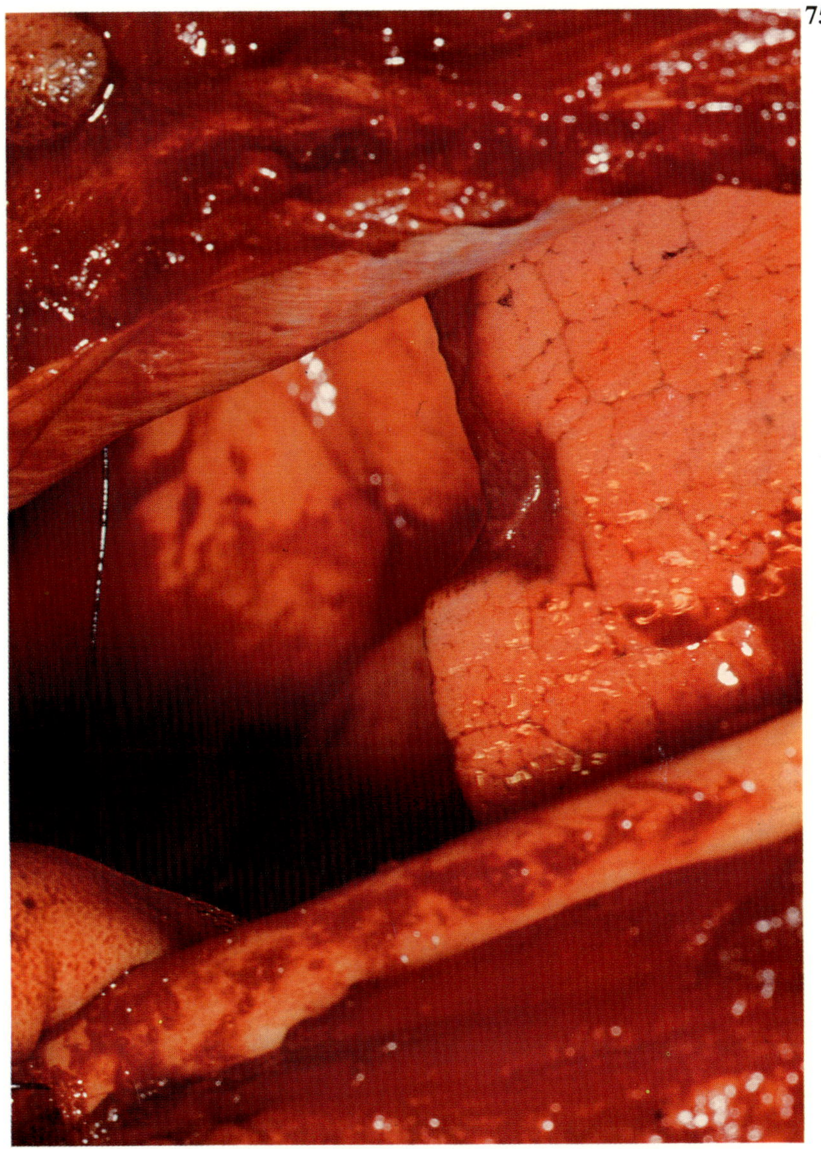

75 Focal collapse. Areas of focal collapse can easily be missed and they may act as a nidus for postoperative infection. Once the surgeon is sure that all areas are inflated a final check should be made for escaping air or any other evidence of damage to the lung. If a laceration of the lung is found it should be sutured with catgut, unless it is very small, and the suture line made as airtight as possible.

76

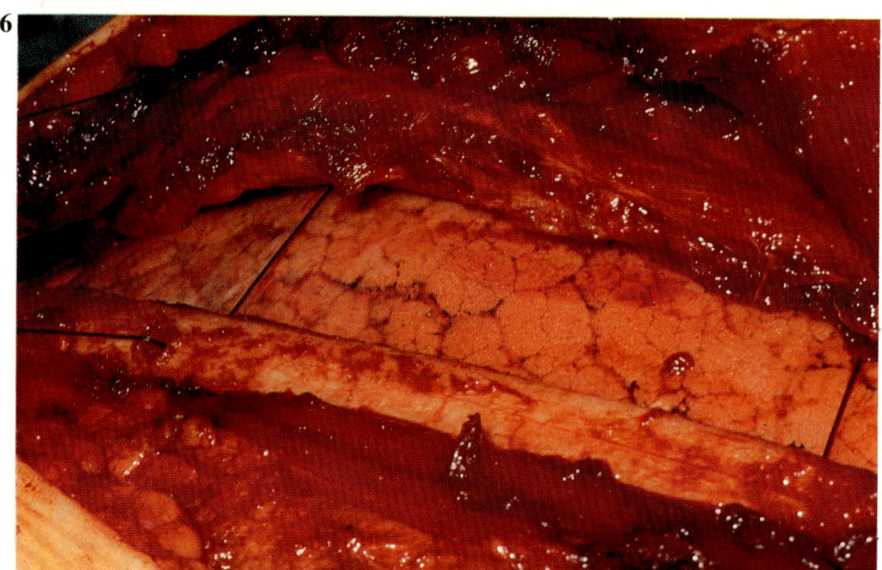

77

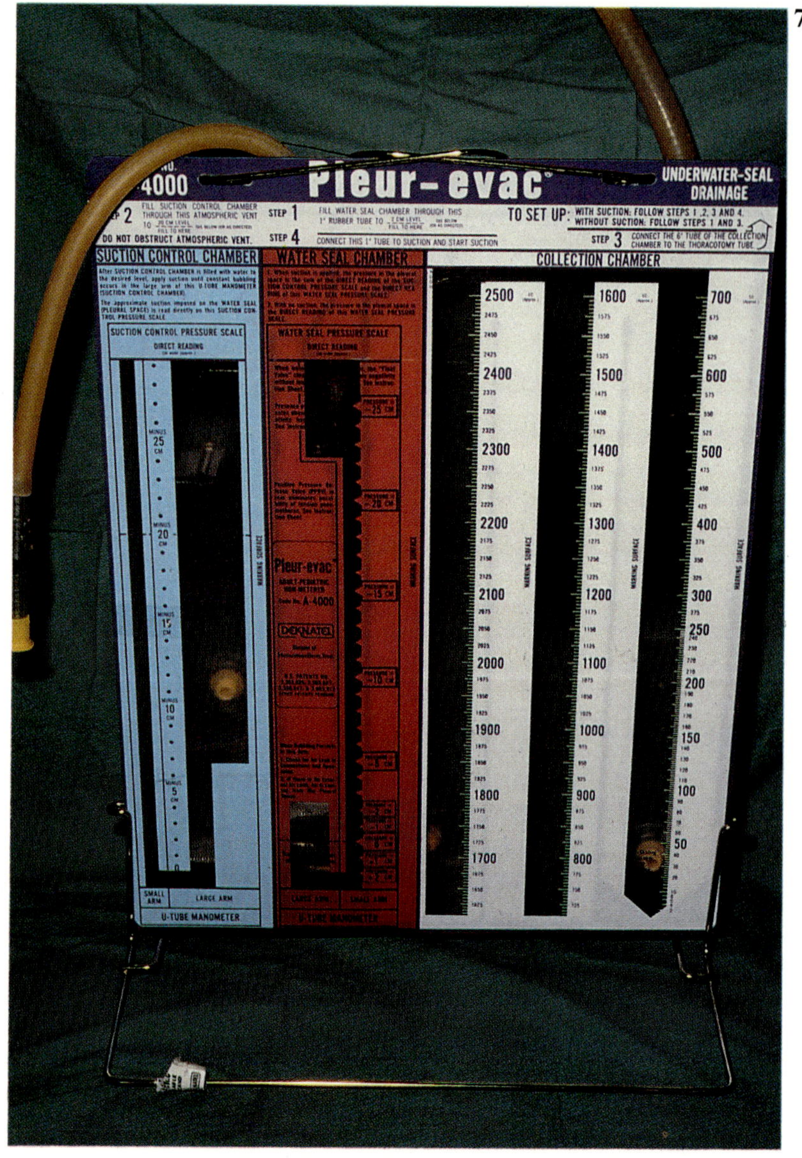

76 Full inflation. The lung is fully inflated and the pleural cavity can now be closed. If an intercostal block is desired, Marcaine is injected into the subcoastal groove at the posterior end of the interspace and also the interspaces above and below—(see page 7).

77 Underwater seal drainage. The chest drain is now connected to some form of underwater seal drainage. The usual, and the cheapest, system is the Winchester bottle. The author prefers the 'Pleur-evac' system for several reasons: the instructions are easy to follow and are on the apparatus; the whole system comes complete with tubing ready for connection; the Pleur-evac can be hung from the bed or mounted on the metal stand shown in the illustration; the amount of discharge from the thorax can be measured with ease; there is usually no need to change the system before the chest drain is removed; negative suction can be applied where necessary without adding extra bottles; and finally it is safer than the bottle system as it is much less likely to be knocked over.
The underwater seal is in the red chamber of the apparatus, the drainage from the thorax is collected in the white chamber and if negative suction is required it takes place in the blue chamber.

78 Pleur-evac instructions. The top part of the apparatus is visualised here to show the instructions, which are given to set the system up with or without suction. They are easily and safely followed.

78

79 Fixation of ribs. The rib approximator is used to bring together the ribs adjacent to the incision and the rib stitches are tied. Once the knots are secure the approximator can be removed.

79

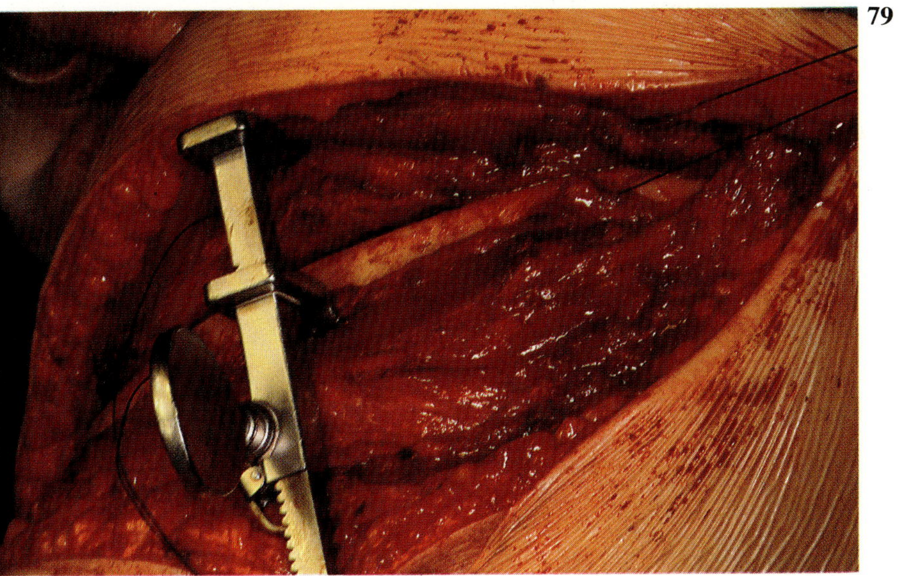

80 Closure of muscle. The author leaves the intercostal muscles unsutured but some surgeons make an attempt to approximate the periosteal flaps which were fashioned when the incision was made. A monofilament nylon suture is inserted in serratus anterior at the posterior end of the wound.

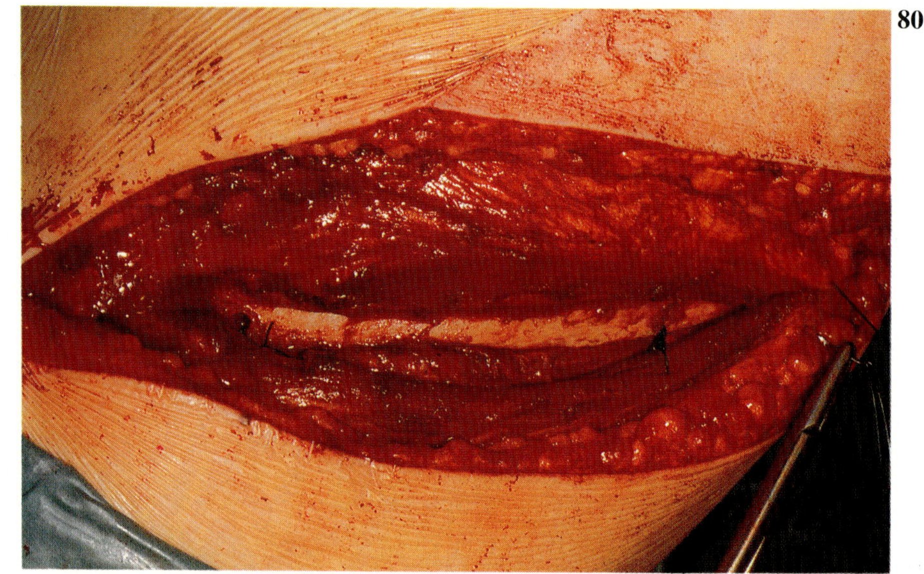

80

81 Serratus and external oblique. This suture is inserted in a continuous fashion and as it moves anteriorly it leaves serratus and picks up external oblique which interdigitates with serratus anterior.

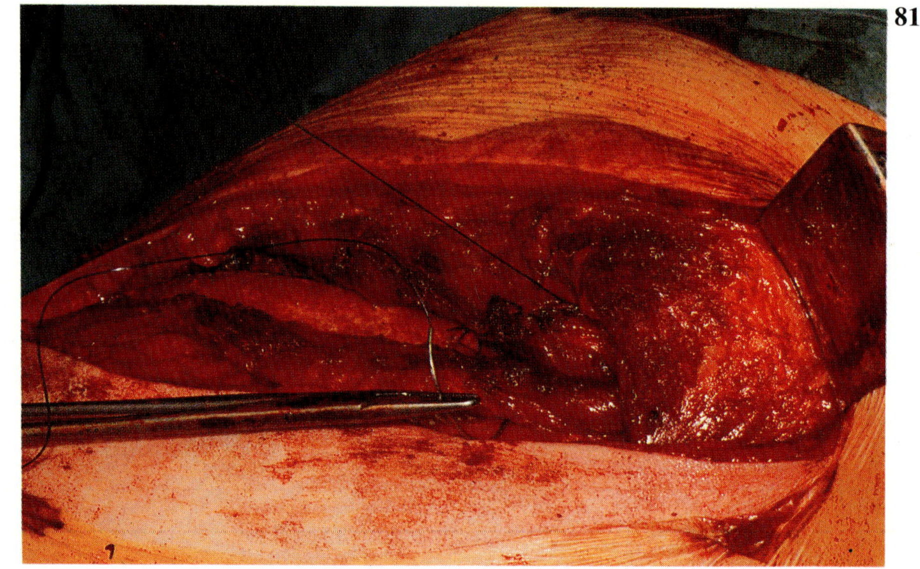

81

82 Latissimus dorsi. A second layer of continuous suture using monofilament nylon is used to close latissimus dorsi and passes forward when it leaves the muscle to close the deep fascia.

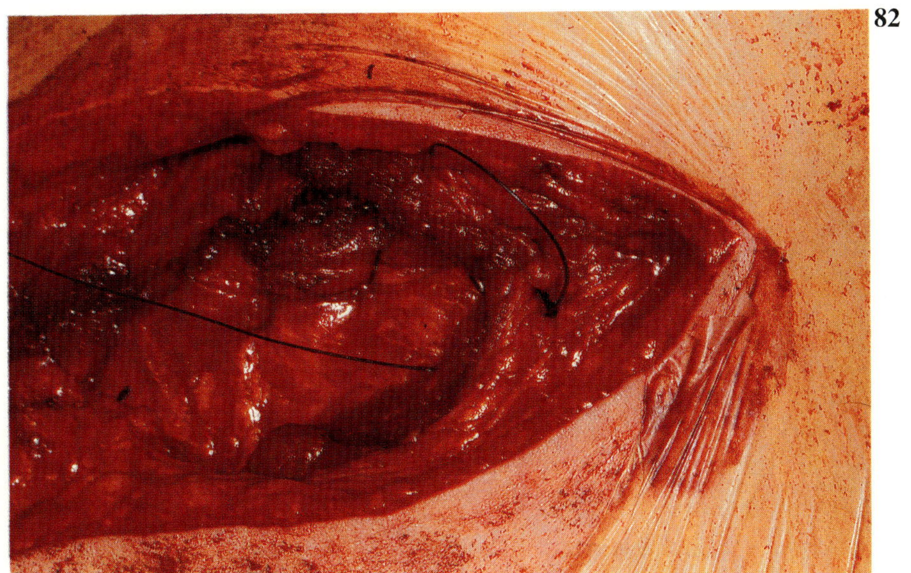

82

83 Mass closure. The author prefers to close each layer separately but mass closure of all muscle in a single layer is becoming popular and this is shown here. Although the author uses nonabsorbable suture material, some surgeons prefer to close with chromic catgut throughout.

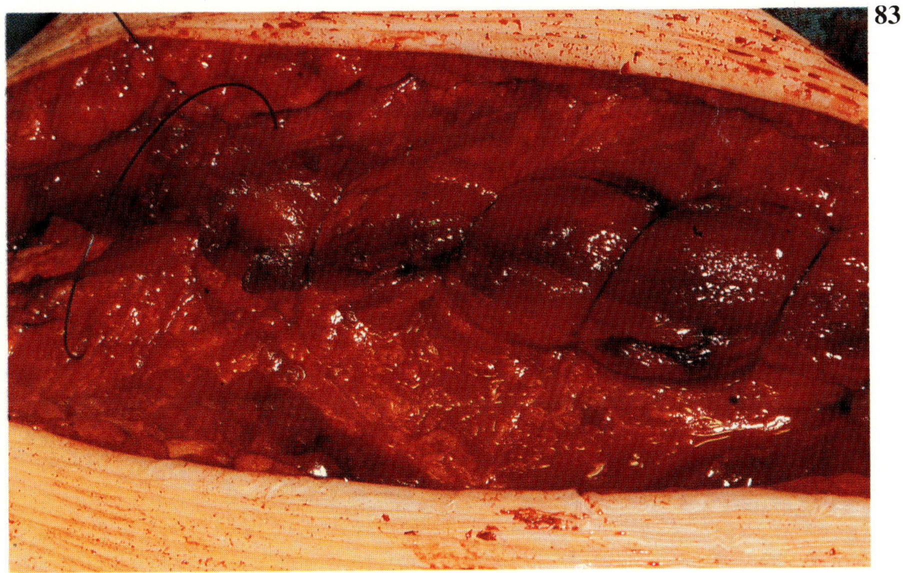

83

84 Final check of lung inflation. The plastic sheet is peeled off the edges of the incision prior to closure of the skin. During the latter part of the closure of the incision, when the surgeon judges that the closure is airtight, the anaesthetist proceeds to 'bag' the patient to express as much air as possible out of the pleural cavity. When this has been done the Pleur-evac is inspected to make sure that the water seal chamber water level is oscillating freely.

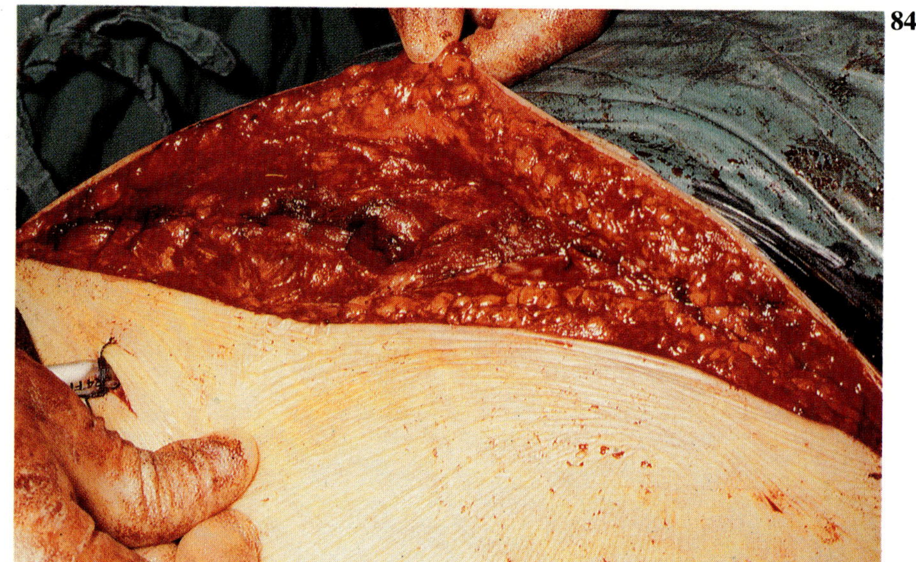
84

85 Cleaning wound edges. The wound edges are cleaned with Savlon and the skin is ready for suturing.

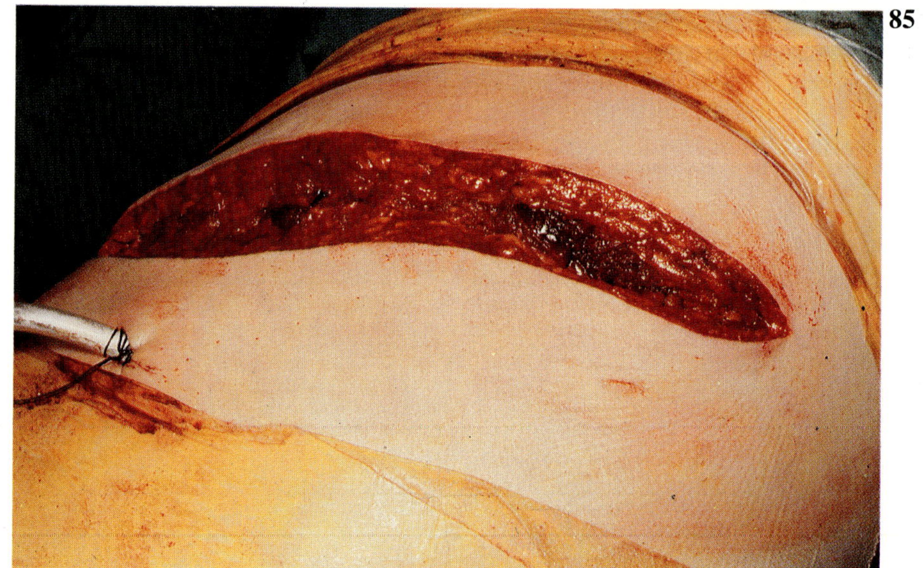
85

86 Skin closure. Many different types of stitch can be used to close the skin but the author prefers a continuous suture such as the subcuticular, which is fashioned with Prolene on a straight needle. This enables good skin apposition without the extrusion of subcutaneous fat which sometimes occurs between badly placed interrupted sutures. A continuous mattress suture or a blanket stitch are other frequently-used methods of closure.

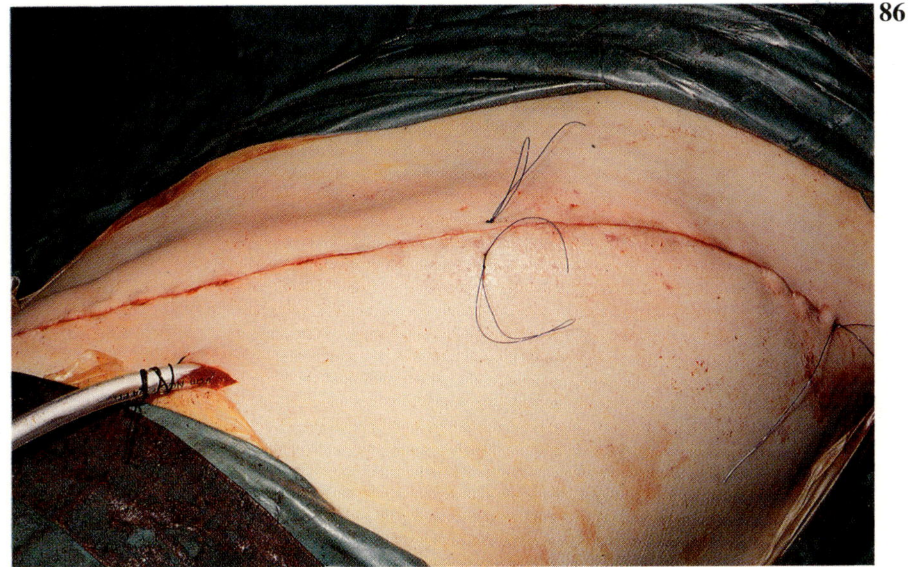

86

87 Wound dressing. The wound dressing consists of many pieces of wound gauze laid along the incision and held in place with an appropriate adhesive dressing. If possible an airtight dressing should be used but often sensitivity of the patient to some of the commercially available adhesive dressings prevents this. Micropore surgical adhesive tape is claimed to be suitable for sensitive individuals.

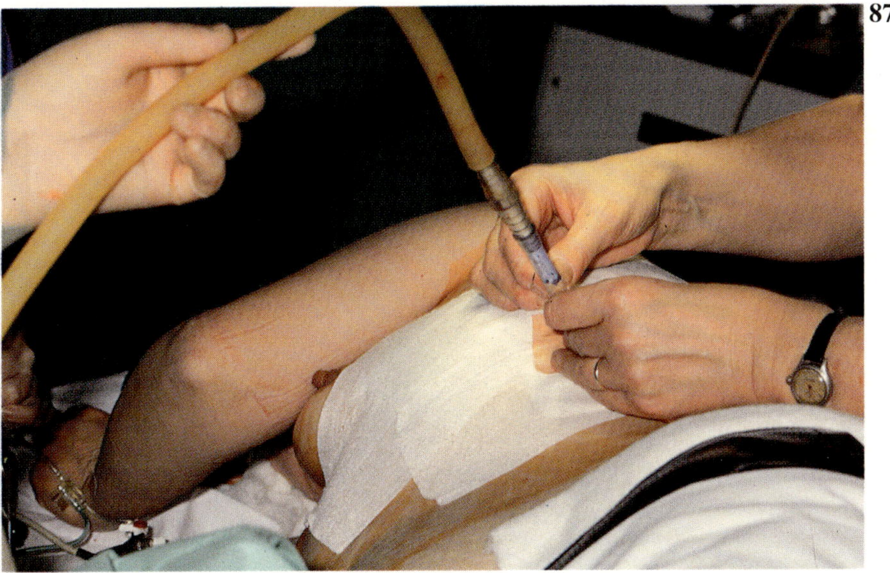

87

88 Securing chest catheter. The chest drain should be firmly fixed as it emerges from the wound dressing and a sound method of achieving this is depicted using two short lengths of Sleek impermeable surgical plastic adhesive tape pressed together with the catheter sandwiched between them.

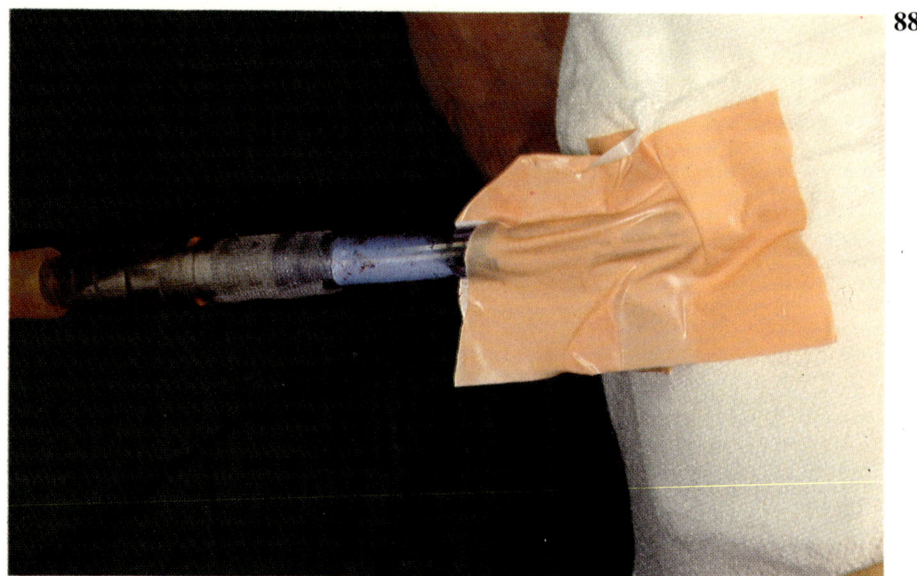

88

89 Sleek adhesive tape. Where no problem exists as far as wound tape sensitivity is concerned Sleek adhesive tape can be used throughout. Only one further small length is necessary to complete the wound dressing and make it as airtight as possible.

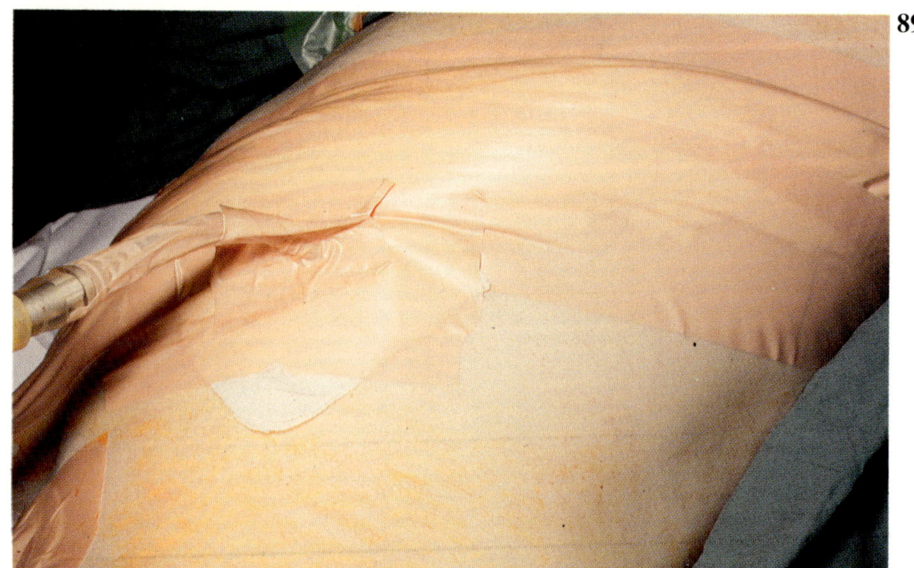

89

Usual postoperative course

The patient should have a chest xray in the recovery area in the immediate postoperative period to make sure that the left lung is fully inflated. The control of pain should be as described in the anaesthetic management section—see pages 7 and 8. The patient is usually sitting up in a chair on the morning after operation for a short period and this period is gradually increased until he begins to walk about after removal of the chest drain.

Physiotherapy is begun as soon as the patient can co-operate and is continued as long as is necessary. **Patient compliance with the physiotherapist is much better if preoperative physiotherapy instruction has been given. Intensive physiotherapy may sometimes be required where there is excessive sputum retention**.

A chest xray is taken on the morning following operation and if there are no problems as regards excessive pleural effusion, collapse, consolidation or pneumothorax the chest drain is clamped for a few hours. If no distress develops the chest drain is removed and the purse string suture is tied. A final chest xray is usually taken on the day following the removal of the drain.

Clear fluid (25 ml) is given orally a few hours after operation and if there is no excessive aspirate, this quantity is stepped up to 50 ml hourly on day 2 and 100 ml hourly on day 3. When this volume of oral fluids has been achieved the intravenous drip can be discontinued and diet commenced. The patient's activity is now gradually increased and he can be allowed home any time after the sixth or seventh postoperative day.

Postoperative complications

The immediate postoperative complications are those of any major thoracic operation and need no special mention here. **The commonest troublesome complication is post-thoracotomy pain and this may require referral of the patient to an anaesthetic colleague with an interest in pain management**. Even in severe cases the condition usually settles completely in time. A few patients complain of slight dysphagia in the early postoperative period but this usually settles spontaneously but may on occasions require a dilatation.

Residual symptoms occur in about 10% of patients and a few of these will ultimately show radiological or endoscopic evidence (or both) of recurrence of the hernia and oesophagitis. **Where the residual symptoms are due to a definite recurrence of the hernia, reoperation may be advised**. **For those patients with residual symptoms but with no evidence of recurrence or reflux the management is much more difficult and reoperation should be avoided**.

Occasionally, if the operation has not been done early enough before serious damage to the oesophageal mucosa has been caused by reflux oesophagitis, a stricture may still develop and bouginage may be required.

Results

Postoperative review is at the surgeon's discretion but unless there is any problem with post-thoracotomy pain, the patient can sleep flat and bend over without reflux by the time of follow-up a few weeks after operation.

The long-term results are well documented and over 90% of patients are very satisfied with the operation. It is very gratifying to see patients, who have been severely disabled with postural dyspepsia, able to stoop and to lie flat without discomfort and who are relieved of disabling indigestion and the sequelae of uncontrolled reflux.

The author and many other surgeons are indebted to Mr Belsey for his pioneering work in the field of hiatus hernia and reflux oesophagitis which led to the development of this effective operation. Where a precise and accurate diagnosis has been made the results are excellent, the recurrence rate is low and its place in the operative management of hiatus hernia is assured.

Further reading

Barish, C.F., Wu, W.C., Castell, D.O. Respiratory complications of gastroesophageal reflux. *Arch Intern Med.,* 1985; **145:** 1882-1892

Baue, A.E. The Belsey Mark V procedure. *Ann. Thorac. Surg.,* 1980; **29:** 265-269

Bennet J.R. Gastro-oesophageal reflux. *Current Opinions in Gasteroenterology,* 1986; **2:** 517-527

Clouse, R.E., Stenson, W.F., Avioli, L.V., Esophageal motility disorders and chest pain. *Arch. Intern. Med.* 1985; **145:** 903-908

Earlam, R., *Clinical Tests of Oesophageal Function.* Crosby Lockwood Staples, London

Evans, D.F., Jones, J.A., Hardcastle, J.D., Ambulatory monitoring of gastro-oesophageal pH using a radiotelemetry capsule and a new solid state recorder with automated analysis. *Gastroenterology,* 1985; **88:** 1376

Hiebert, C.A., O'Mara, C.S., The Belsey operation for hiatal hernia: a twenty-year experience. *Am. J. Surg.,* 1979; **137:** 532

Orringer, M.B., Skinner, D.B., Belsey, R.H.R., Long-term results of the Mark IV operation for hiatal hernia and analysis of recurrences and their treatment. *J. Thorac. Cardiovasc. Surg.,* 1972; **63:** 25-31

Payne, W.S., Olsen, A.M., *The Oesophagus.* Lea and Febiger, 1974, Philadelphia

Singh, S.V., Present concept of the Belsey Mark IV procedure: *gastroesophageal reflux and hiatus hernia. Brit. J. Surg.,* 1980; **67;** 26-28

Skinner, D.B., Belsey, R.H.R., Surgical management of esophageal reflux and hiatus hernia. *J. Thorac. Cardiovasc. Surg.,* 1967; **53:** 33-50

Surgical treatment of hiatus hernia. *Brit. Med. J.,* 1977; **2:** 1437

INDEX

All numbers refer to pages

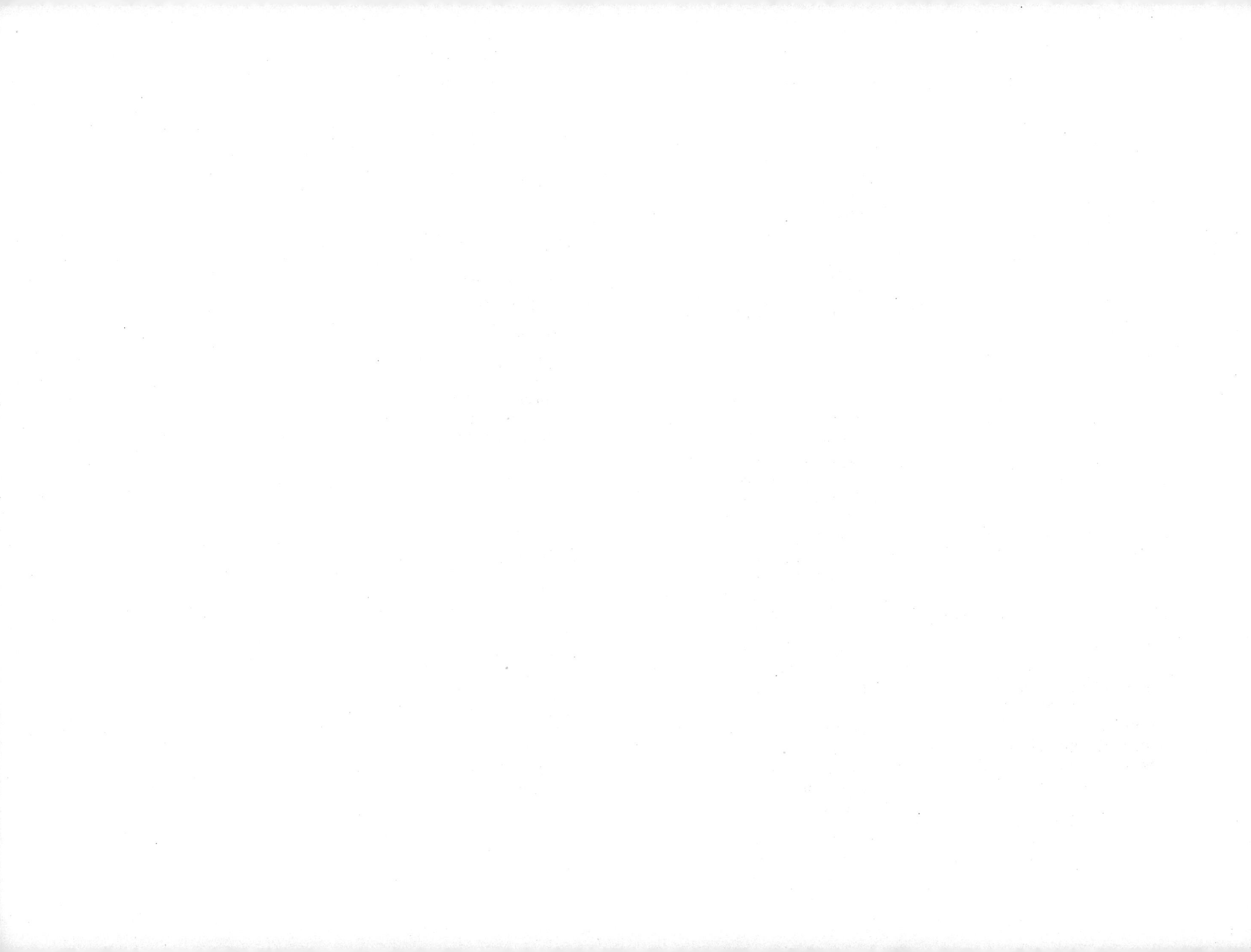